BMA

il

PAIN
AND
PREJUDICE

major contribution to feminist writing of the 21st century. Jackson
kes her own story of endometriosis, a neglected and mistreated
ndition, and builds around it a careful analysis of how women's
n has been ignored or belittled over centuries by a sexist medical
fession. She then turns to recent developments, reporting on
dence-based research that is starting to bring better options to
men experiencing chronic pain. Well written, and sometimes
rious, with excellent chapters on women's anatomy and physiology,
is highly recommended reading for all women, their partners and
nilies—and their doctors.'
ROLINE DE COSTA, **Professor of Obstetrics and Gynaecology,
nes Cook University** i

abrielle Jackson deploys facts to tear away the destructive myths that
rround women's health and to unpick the sexism woven so tightly
o the medical system. On behalf all the women who continue to
fer unnecessarily, she demands change.'
NORE TAYLOR, **Editor,** *Guardian Australia*

his book is a brilliant, blood-drenc
man and man—and most particular
Gabrielle Jackson has made it her
pant ignorance around women and
"normal" part of being alive.'
LY WILSON, **Editor,** *New Scientist*

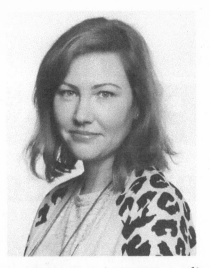

Gabrielle Jackson is an associate news editor at *Guardian Australia*, and was previously opinion editor there. Before that she was a senior journalist at *The Hoopla*. Gabrielle has lived and worked in the USA, UK and Australia as a journalist and copywriter. She currently lives in Sydney and commutes regularly to the Riverina district of New South Wales. Gabrielle was first diagnosed with endometriosis in 2001. In 2015 she was also diagnosed with adenomyosis. After writing about endometriosis for *The Guardian* in 2015, she became interested in how women's pain is treated in modern healthcare systems and has been researching and writing about the topic since then.

Gabrielle loves cooking and is a kebab connoisseur. In 2011–2012, she spent eight months travelling from Europe through the Middle East to Asia researching the history of kebabs and their journey to the western world. She returned to Australia after being run over by a train in India.

A CALL TO ARMS FOR
WOMEN AND THEIR BODIES

PAIN
AND
PREJUDICE

Gabrielle Jackson

piatkus

PIATKUS

First published in Australia in 2019 by Allen & Unwin
First published in Great Britain in 2019 by Piatkus

1 3 5 7 9 10 8 6 4 2

A CIP catalogue record for this book
is available from the British Library.

ISBN 978-0-349-42455-2

Illustrations on pages 21, 22, 33, 37, 40, 48 and 187 by Ngaio Parr Index by Garry Cousins
Set in 13/17.6 pt Bembo by Midland Typesetters, Australia

Printed and bound in Great Britain by Clays Ltd, Elcograf S.p.A

Papers used by Piatkus are from well-managed forests and
other responsible sources.

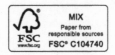

Piatkus
An imprint of
Little, Brown Book Group
Carmelite House
50 Victoria Embankment
London EC4Y 0DZ

An Hachette UK Company
www.hachette.co.uk

www.littlebrown.co.uk

CONTENTS

Introduction   1

1   Repeat after me, *vulva*: the female reproductive
    system   19
2   'Worse than the Loch Ness monster': menstruation
    and menopause   42
3   From clitoridectomy to the talking cure: a history
    of hysteria   80
4   Neither Madonna nor whore: rethinking female
    sexuality   117
5   It's the culture, stupid: understanding modern
    medical practice   158
6   'The pain that can't be seen': a new appreciation
    of women's pain   213
7   Time to ditch the bikini: the women's health
    conditions you never hear about   256
8   'Ripe for disruption': why medical science must
    improve its knowledge of women   292

Epilogue   318
Acknowledgements   322
Notes   324
Index   347

INTRODUCTION

I was watching my young niece's swimming lesson when the familiar pain hit. It began with the usual ache in the gut that travelled down my legs and up my back but became sharp so quickly I doubled over. I felt beads of sweat accumulate at my temples and under my arms. A weakness overcame me and I knew I had to get to the toilet fast. After telling my sister I didn't feel well, I hobbled off to the public bathroom. I didn't have any painkillers on me and the nausea just got worse. I sat on the toilet bent in half at the waist. I had diarrhoea but it didn't make me feel better. I was sweating a lot.

My niece's lesson finished. She and my sister showered, changed, ate a snack and were ready to go. My sister was calling for me. I hobbled out of the cubicle, trying not to worry anyone. I vomited in the carpark and held back tears. The pain was so severe, I could barely talk to answer my sister's questions.

At her place she gave me some painkillers and prepared a hot water bottle for me as I vomited again in the toilet. She rang our mum for advice and kept asking me, 'What can I do?'

But there was nothing she could do. Being at her house was at least better than having to lie down in a public bathroom alone.

Now I never leave home without a bag filled with pain-killers, anti-inflammatories, and drugs to prevent abdominal cramping, nausea and diarrhoea. I've grown used to the sudden onset of overwhelming pain and nausea, and the embarrassment that causes. I've become expert at pinpointing the exact moment I need to get home—when the beads of sweat begin to form at my temples, under my arms and at the base of my spine. Around the same time, a weakness in my legs gives way to stabbing pains in my lower abdomen. When that happens, I know I have half an hour to take some painkillers and anti-nausea drugs, fill a hot water bottle and be still.

If I can't get home in time, things can get ugly.

———

'I have a disease that I know nothing about.
I thought I knew everything, or at least a lot about it—but
that turned out to be very far from the truth and also very
bad for my health.'[1]

That was the first sentence of a feature I wrote for *The Guardian* about having endometriosis. I was 38 and had suffered with various health problems since my teens. I'd always thought of myself as weak; I was jealous of the energy my friends could muster. I knew I had a disease but didn't want to be seen as sick—I didn't want to be a whinger or thought of as no fun. At some point I normalised most of my pain, and I believed my constant back and hip aches were the result of a skiing accident I'd had at nineteen.

But if I was cursed with endometriosis, I was blessed with a cheery disposition and an almost pathological optimism. This enabled the central paradox of my life. I was never one to suffer in silence; people close to me knew of my ongoing physical ailments while having little comprehension of their emotional toll. Like me, my loved ones didn't ascribe all my loud complaints to the burden of a chronic disease. I gave myself the title of hypochondriac before it could become a complaint whispered behind my back.

I lived in cycles. For months at a time I'd be incredibly busy with work and social commitments, then I'd become exhausted: in intense physical pain, emotional and always on the verge of tears. During these periods, I locked myself away at home, took long baths and lots of painkillers, and fortified my body and mind for the next cycle. My only excuse was, 'I'm just so tired.'

After one particularly bad flare-up—in which I'd spent the 2014 Christmas holiday period in bed with my best friend, the hot water bottle—I heard about a patient-centred endometriosis conference run by the advocacy group EndoActive. I got myself a ticket.

One crisp day the following May in a University of Sydney auditorium, I learnt for the first time that all the things wrong with me—the period pain, leg pain, back pain, hip pain, shooting pains up my rectum and vagina, bloating, nausea, diarrhoea, stomach upsets, dizziness, and the oh-so-debilitating fatigue—were common symptoms of endometriosis. I also heard of adenomyosis for the first time, a disease I was diagnosed with later that year. I cried and I cried and I cried. For most of my life I'd doubted myself, feeling second-rate, weak and flaky, only to realise . . . I wasn't. I had to reimagine myself, and it wasn't easy.

I told my editor at *The Guardian*, Emily Wilson (now editor of *New Scientist*), I wanted to write about endometriosis. She could barely believe the statistics: one in ten women of reproductive age have the disease. That's 176 million women worldwide. Sufferers are routinely told by healthcare professionals that pregnancy or hysterectomy are cures—they're not. In fact, there's no known cause or cure.

Medical professionals often dismiss sufferers as being difficult rather than ill. One gynaecologist wrote about how the disease can be cured by stress management because only type A personalities get it. Another gynaecologist wondered aloud to a researcher, 'Do mad people get endo or does endo make you mad?' 'It's probably a bit of both,' he concluded. An anaesthetist told a pain seminar that women with treatment-resistant endo have probably been sexually abused and need to see a psychiatrist. The disease is funded at around 5 per cent of the rate of funding for diabetes although it affects about the same number of women and costs the economy more; and the personal financial cost is exorbitant—unlike for diabetes, which has many affordable treatment options. Figures in 2018 were remarkably similar in Australia, the US and UK.

My editor was shocked. She consulted *The Guardian*'s editor-in-chief, Katharine Viner, and the best health reporters from *The Guardian*'s global team were recruited to do an investigation. It happened swiftly and efficiently, and I was blown away by the result.

When we asked endo sufferers to tell us about their experiences on 10 September 2015, we received more than 600 responses in under 24 hours. We had to close the submission form because we couldn't possibly publish them all. As I was reading through the stories, one thing became clear to me: no matter their country, ethnicity or race, or how old, rich or poor, sufferers from around the world faced the same battles: long delays in diagnosis, having their pain doubted then normalised, having their mental health questioned and receiving bad medical advice. (There was even one Russian woman who'd been given leech therapy—a trend I'd assumed had been discredited a couple of centuries ago but may apparently be making a comeback!) The quality-of-life impact was extreme for women who responded from Australia, the UK, Ireland, the USA, Canada, Uganda, Armenia, Brazil, Poland, Nepal and Thailand. The financial cost along with the costs of opportunities lost in school, at work and in relationships are untold.

Endometriosis has been known as the 'silent disease', but that isn't because women don't want to talk about it. On 28 September 2015 when *The Guardian* launched its global investigation into endometriosis,[2] a million people clicked; my feature alone has been shared more than 40,000 times. Everywhere I went in the weeks following that investigation, people wanted to talk about endo with me. I received hundreds of emails—and more than three years later, I'm still getting emails from women who relate to my story. So many of them tell me it feels like I found *their* words, because their story is frighteningly similar to mine. We're linked only by our experiences with an insidious disease, one that's common yet ignored, and with a worldwide patriarchal healthcare system.

A DAWNING REALISATION

I've been diagnosed with two diseases of the reproductive organs. Endometriosis is a chronic inflammatory disease in which tissue similar to the lining of the uterus, known as the endometrium, grows in other parts of the body, most commonly the pelvic cavity. Adenomyosis is when endometrium-like tissue grows inside the muscle wall of the uterus. One gynaecologist told me that my only option was to have a hysterectomy; another told me this was rubbish.

I decided to learn everything I could about the two diseases— and the more research I did, the more enraged I became at medical professionals, research organisations, pharmaceutical companies, governments and policy-makers. I realised endometriosis and adenomyosis weren't the only diseases largely being ignored—this was the norm for almost any illness affecting women in particular. And I'm not just talking about conditions of the reproductive system, such as endometriosis, pelvic pain and polycystic ovaries. It's any condition that, for some reason, mostly women get or that reacts differently in women than men. Let me give you three examples.

Heart disease

I'm starting with the big one: heart disease is the leading cause of death among women globally. It has traditionally been thought of as a man's disease, which has led to deadly consequences for women—in 2004, 7.4 million women over 60 years of age died of cardiovascular disease compared with 6.3 million men.[3]

Almost everything known about heart disease and its treatments has been learnt from studying men, so doctors have been trained to recognise the signs and symptoms of heart attacks, cardiovascular conditions and strokes in men. But heart disease can work differently in women to men. Australian cardiothoracic surgeon Dr Nikki Stamp spends a big part of her spare time trying to raise awareness about heart disease in women; she tells me, 'There's this difference in biology between a man's heart attack and a woman's heart attack. What this means is that the symptoms can be different, our diagnostic tests may not be geared to pick up the problem and also our treatments probably don't work as well for that different biology.' When sufferers present with so-called atypical symptoms—typical in women, just not in men—they're often misdiagnosed or sent home with anxiety. A 2018 study published in the *Medical Journal of Australia* found that women were half as likely to be treated properly for a heart attack as men and twice as likely to die six months after discharge.[4] A 2017 US study found that only 22 per cent of primary-care physicians and 42 per cent of cardiologists said they felt extremely well prepared to assess women's cardiovascular risk.[5]

Many women don't know they're at risk, delay seeking treatment because they think they can't be affected, and don't recognise their symptoms as heart disease. Women who have pre-eclampsia, gestational diabetes or high blood pressure during pregnancy are at particular risk for cardiovascular disease and stroke, yet many are not aware.

A 2017 University of Sydney study published in *Heart* found that women were 12 per cent less likely than men to have cardiovascular disease risk factors such as smoking status, blood pressure and total cholesterol measured during medical consultations.[6]

Autoimmune conditions

Autoimmune conditions affect between 5 and 10 per cent of the global population. They occur when our immune system, which defends the body against bacteria, viruses and other germs, turns on itself and starts to attack its own healthy cells, tissues or organs. These conditions are estimated to cost society between US$80 and $100 billion annually.[7] And yet, medical science is virtually ignorant of their causes, and there are no cures for the 100-odd autoimmune conditions that we know of.

Women account for three-quarters of people with auto-immune conditions, a leading cause of death and disability. While this disparity has been evident for well over a hundred years, only this century has attention started to focus on sex and gender differences in autoimmune diseases. We now know that men and women experience different basic immune responses: women's are more vigorous and make more anti-bodies. Some scientists believe this more flexible immune system is responsible for women's longer life spans—it seems women survive some infections that would kill men.

But women around the world face lengthy delays in diag-nosis for autoimmune conditions. Almost half the women eventually diagnosed with one of these diseases will have been told by doctors that they're hypochondriacs or 'too concerned with their health'.[8] Many will first be diagnosed with a mental illness, and while depression is a common symptom of auto-immune conditions, it's rarely treated as part of the whole condition: no single medical speciality covers all functions affected by autoimmune disease.

You could call the female immune system women's

kryptonite—the very source of our greatest strength, survival, is also the cause of our greatest weakness, illness.

Chronic pain

Women experience more chronic pain than men, and the disparity lasts through their entire reproductive lives. As children, boys and girls experience roughly the same levels of pain, but once girls reach adolescence, the number of them experiencing pain that lasts more than three months—known as chronic pain—is leaps and bounds ahead of the number of boys.

Almost all the major chronic pain conditions affect more women than men, including endometriosis and vulvodynia, obviously, but also rheumatoid arthritis, migraines and temporomandibular joint disorders. And scientists have now discovered that chronic pain works differently in male versus female brains, which is a problem because almost all the pain research has traditionally been done using male cell lines, and male rodent and human participants.

Then there are the 'contested' chronic pain conditions, such as fibromyalgia, chronic fatigue syndrome/myalgic encephalomyelitis, irritable bowel syndrome and interstitial cystitis/painful bladder syndrome. Not only do doctors not agree on names for some of these conditions—hence the slashes—they can't even agree that they exist. It's no coincidence that women outnumber men in all of these conditions. Patients suffer from delays in diagnosis (often after misdiagnoses), having their symptoms dismissed and disbelieved, and being diagnosed with mental health conditions.

While chronic pain affects the same number of people as cancer, heart disease and diabetes combined, it receives 95 per cent less research funding in the United States, with similar discrepancies worldwide.[9] The historic report, *Relieving Pain in America*,[10] found that four in ten adults live with chronic pain disorders, and recognised a cluster of pain conditions that frequently co-occur solely or predominantly in women. These were later given a term by the US Congress, 'chronic over-lapping pain conditions'. The Chronic Pain Research Alliance was formed to advocate on behalf of the people affected by these ten conditions—endometriosis, vulvodynia, fibromy-algia, chronic fatigue syndrome/myalgic encephalomyelitis, interstitial cystitis/painful bladder syndrome, temporoman-dibular joint disorders, irritable bowel syndrome, chronic tension-type headache, chronic migraine and chronic low back pain—all of which are beset by misdiagnosis, lack of coordinated medical care and a sparsity of safe and effective treatment options.

SO WHY AREN'T WOMEN GETTING THE DEAL WE DESERVE?

For too long, women's longer life spans have obscured the real picture of women's health. Because the truth is this: although women live longer, they live fewer healthy active years than men. Women are in pain, all through their bodies; they're in pain with their periods, and while having sex; they have pelvic pain, migraine, headaches, joint aches, painful bladders, irritable bowels, sore lower backs, muscle pain, vulval pain, vaginal pain, jaw pain, muscle aches. And many are so, so tired. Women are diagnosed with depression, anxiety, post-traumatic stress disorder and behavioural personality disorder at much higher rates than men.

But women's pain is all too often dismissed, their illnesses misdiagnosed or ignored. Women are treated as unreliable witnesses to their own health, while diseases that mainly affect them are under-researched; even when it comes to diseases that affect both women and men, symptoms and treatments are mainly studied in men, which leads to misdiagnosis and under-treatment in women.

In medicine, man is the default human being. Any deviation is atypical, abnormal, deficient.

WHY DO WE LIVE LIKE THIS?

Many factors are at play, but it all comes down to this: a world controlled by men. In this book I'm focusing on three main issues in trying to understand why we are where we are—and what needs to change so we can fix this situation.

Education and taboos

The first part of this book looks at women's lack of education on how our bodies work, and social taboos and stigmas that prevent many women from talking about our genitals, sex life, pain and reproductive processes. How can we talk about pain that's sexual or focused on our reproductive organs, when we don't even know the names for parts of our anatomy?

The Eve Appeal, a British gynaecological cancer charity, found that 44 per cent of women couldn't correctly identify a vagina in a diagram and 15 per cent wouldn't consult a doctor about a lump in their vagina.[11] These results help show how pervasive the taboos around women's health are, and how these societal norms rule—and ruin—even the most modern lives. They also show how much work has to be done to break these taboos. For better or worse, women can't do that alone.

'When we ignore the body, we are more easily victimised by it,' wrote Milan Kundera in *The Unbearable Lightness of Being*. Women's general ignorance about our bodies doesn't seem to have arisen by accident but rather by design. Why aren't school-children taught the correct names for female anatomy? Why is menstruation a topic that must be discussed in hushed tones? And the myths around menopause are so perverse, one expert compared them to those surrounding the Loch Ness monster.[12]

Hysteria and modern medical practice

To understand how women are treated by the healthcare profession today, we must first understand how they were treated in the past. For most of human history, the widespread idea that a woman is inherently irrational and brimming with uncontrollable emotions and bodily functions has justified her subordination—kept her in the home, and locked her out of education and professional careers. From the birth of medicine in ancient times until the modern era, the womb was blamed for almost any illness that befell women, many of them gathered under the label 'hysteria'; then, around a century ago, hormones came to be seen as the major culprit.

Hysteria, a disease widely recognised by Western doctors from the seventeenth until the twentieth century, was char-acterised by symptoms that enigmatically changed over time. The condition was originally thought to be a physical disease caused by the womb, and brutal surgeries were performed in efforts to cure it. Later, Freud and others helped popular-ise the notion that hysteria was all in the mind. At its root, hysteria has always been about women's pain—and medicine's failure to deal with it—and her sexuality, as well as prevailing social conditions. While the word 'hysteria' eventually disappeared from medical textbooks, its legend lives on in how doctors respond to women with complex problems that they don't have answers for. Medical practitioners aren't well trained to deal with conditions for which knowledge is scarce. They receive little training in treating patients with chronic diseases that have few treatment options, and they're effectively taught to blame the patient if she's a woman who doesn't get well or they can't diagnose her symptoms. Dr Kate Young from Melbourne's Monash University has studied notions of hysteria in the treatment of endometriosis. She found that while doctors don't necessarily hold sexist views, when a woman continues to complain after all the available treatment tools have been exhausted, it's at this stage that hysteria narratives start to emerge. Doctors tend to believe that since they have done everything they can to help the patient, it must be something she is doing that stops her feeling well: she's not following advice, it's her lifestyle choices, or she has a mental illness that is making her believe she's ill when she's not.

Medicine has even dreamt up a new illness—'medically unexplained symptoms'—that has deep connotations of hysteria, hypochondria and attention-seeking. And what's one of the major risk factors for 'medically unexplained symptoms'? Being a woman.

Scientific research

When doctors dredge up hysteria narratives to explain women with symptoms they can't cure, they fail to acknowledge the fundamental truth of medical science: it simply doesn't know much about women.

In 1990, the US National Institutes of Health (NIH), the world's largest medical research body, formed the Office of Research on Women's Health in response to a campaign to include more women in clinical trials. The office's first agenda-setting paper in 1991 noted a 'pervasive sense in the research community that many of the health issues of women are of secondary importance, especially those that occur solely in women and those that occur in men and women but have already been studied chiefly in men'.[13] More than two decades later, Dr Janine Austin Clayton, the current director of this office, told the *New York Times*, 'We literally know less about every aspect of female biology compared to male biology.'[14] This is supported by something that Dr Nanette Wenger, a leading US heart disease expert, wrote in 2004: 'The medical community has viewed women's health with a bikini approach, focusing essentially on the breast and reproductive system. The rest of the woman was virtually ignored in considerations of women's health.'[15]

This attitude helps explain why medicine knows very little about conditions that mainly affect women, and also why women receive worse outcomes in cardiovascular diseases. Finding treatments would involve looking for them, something that hasn't ever been a priority for medical science.

Let's look again at chronic pain. Currently, 70 per cent of chronic-pain patients are women but 80 per cent of pain studies are conducted on men or male mice.[16] Only since 2016 has the NIH ruled that pain drugs must be tested in female rodents as well as males. What the NIH decides influences research around the world and funding bodies in Western nations have followed suit with similar rules. One pain researcher, Professor Mark Hutchinson, who has worked in the US and Australia, told me how his team in the US created female-like pain in male rodents just by transferring a type of immune cell called microglia from females into males.[17] This discovery could have profound effects on research and treatment development, and, hopefully, medical practice. Hutchinson is almost certain that some treatment ideas were thrown into the scientific wastebasket because they didn't work on men but could potentially change the lives of women.

WHY DID I WRITE THIS BOOK?

Women wait longer for pain medication than men,[18] are more likely to have their physical symptoms ascribed to mental health issues,[19] and are more likely to have their heart disease misdiagnosed,[20] become disabled after a stroke,[21] suffer from illnesses ignored or denied by the medical profession, and wait longer to be diagnosed for cancer.[22]

I discovered all these facts after I decided to do some research into the two diseases I had been diagnosed with. I was shocked. I wanted to know why women weren't being treated better, why diseases that affect us are ignored or belittled, and I wanted to know why more people weren't talking about all these shocking facts.

I started out being quite angry at doctors who had misdiagnosed or dismissed me but I soon realised that the situation we're in isn't because of a few doctors being sexist. Like many examples of shocking sexism, the problem is structural and not easy to solve. A widespread lack of medical knowledge about women's health is buoyed by a society that makes a taboo of women discussing their problems, especially those to do with reproductive organs. Women aren't supposed to enjoy sex, much less talk about it. Women are supposed to have pain but suffer in silence, then become invisible after menopause. We aren't supposed to be angry, or demand answers. We are supposed to be nice. Put up with it. Be quiet and supportive of others.

When women have the symptoms of our physical illnesses ignored, and when we get angry about it, we're diagnosed with mental illnesses. This helps support and prolong the idea of the hysterical woman. But medical science is an extraordinary force, capable of making great strides in short periods, and it's the best hope women have of getting better. Over the past four years, I've met countless doctors and researchers, male and female, who are working passionately to help improve the lives of women.

Full disclosure: my partner is a male doctor and my mother was a nurse, so I have a soft spot for the profession. But I've met too many women who tell horror stories of their interactions with doctors to ignore the fact that there are still many doctors out there who don't believe it's their job to listen to women—who still believe women's natural state is to be in pain, and they should just shut up and put up with it. What this disguises is the fact that doctors are ill-equipped to treat women's pain, that they haven't been trained to acknowledge when they don't have answers, and that the system in which they work is hostile to treating women—and patients in general—with complex problems.

Like all institutions, medicine is hard to change from the

inside. Major advancements are often prompted by outside efforts, such as when patient groups place so much pressure on governments that they find the money to make developing treatments a priority—this was certainly the case with fighting both breast cancer and HIV/AIDS. Medical science can help us, but first it needs us to shout very loudly. In a 2014 documentary called *Endo What?*, filmmaker and endometriosis patient Shannon Cohn interviews the president of the US-based Endometriosis Association, Mary Lou Ballweg, about why there is such a lack of knowledge about, and effective treatments available for, endometriosis. Ballweg, who has been a campaigner, researcher and advocate for women with endo for 40 years, says, 'Until the group that is affected stands up and says, "Enough already!" it will not stop.'

This book is my way of saying, 'Enough.'

A NOTE ON LANGUAGE

I am a cisgender woman—that means I was born with female sex organs, was raised as a girl and identify as a woman.

There's a difference between sex and gender. Sex relates to common biological differences between males and females, specifically in the sex organs and genetic markers. Gender relates to social norms, and the roles males and females are expected to fulfil as well as one's own gender identity.

There are many people who have female sex organs, who menstruate, who suffer from endometriosis, adenomyosis, and many of the other conditions discussed in this book, who are not women, or do not identify as women.

Where possible I've tried to use inclusive language so as not to exclude these people from my book or erase their experiences. However, pain is a gendered issue. These conditions are under-researched, under-funded and largely unacknowledged because they solely or predominantly affect women. The vast majority of people affected are women. Sadly, most research still fails to distinguish between sex and gender, which makes it all the more difficult for me to draw out conclusions beyond cisgender women.

I've looked for research into trans*, intersex and gender non-binary people's experiences of medicine when dealing with the conditions that I talk about in this book. Unfortunately, the research is still scarce, but I did see signs of hope for the future and have tried to include what research I found.

However, because of the lack of research and the historical treatment of women that has influenced modern medical science and practice, much of this book is about the experiences of cisgender women, and I frequently use the term 'women' to reflect that.

CHAPTER 1

Repeat after me, *vulva*: the female reproductive system

Do you know when you ovulate? Do you know how many eggs are in your ovaries? Do you know how many days a month you're fertile, or what the fallopian tubes do, or the cervix, or the endometrium? Could you point to the labia majora on a diagram? What about the clitoris? Speaking of the clitoris, do you know how many nerve endings it has?

Don't worry, you're not alone. Until I went to that Endo-Active conference a few years ago, I was shockingly ignorant of the basic functions of my body—what's worse, I didn't know it.

When I was asked by my gynaecologist if my endometriosis caused ovulation pain—a symptom I'd never heard of before—I was on the contraceptive pill. I reported that it didn't, without knowing you don't ovulate when you're on the pill. I thought I was lucky not to be one of those poor women cursed with ovulation pain, fatigue and bloating . . . until I stopped taking the pill.

I was trying to get pregnant, so at the chemist I bought a very sophisticated ('99 per cent accurate') ovulation kit that involved me peeing on a stick to determine the best times to have sex. Something funny happened: I noticed that on the days when the test line on the stick was boldest, showing I was about to ovulate, I had cramps, and I often had a headache and felt quite tired. After a few months, I realised that the extraordinary bloating I showed off as a sneak preview to what I'd look like at five months pregnant was also linked to ovulation. The spotting I often had, which I'd thought was irregular bleeding, wasn't irregular at all: ovulation bleeding is a common phenomenon.

After a while, I didn't need the stick to know I was ovulating. It would start with a small throbbing pain in one side of my lower abdomen. Headaches would follow. I was tired. It wasn't too much to deal with but I learnt to get in early with the ibuprofen and schedule some early nights.

The Germans have a name for ovulation pain: mittelschmerz. Literally this translates as 'middle pain', and it's the medical term applied to ovulation pain or middle-cycle pain. I once heard a doctor remark that 'they' don't know if mittelschmerz is really a 'thing'. Well, now I've been off any hormonal medication for more than two years, I can tell any doctor willing to listen: 'Yes, it's a thing.'

That Milan Kundera line keeps going through my head: 'When we ignore the body, we are more easily victimised by it.'

So let's start here: this is a picture of the female reproductive system. Can you name each part?

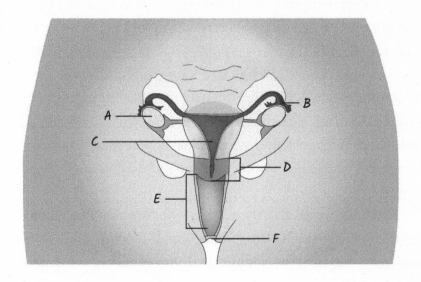

A 2016 UK survey[1] found that fewer than a third of women were able to correctly identify six labelled parts on a diagram of the female reproductive system. Almost half of women (44 per cent) couldn't correctly point out the vagina, and a whopping 60 per cent couldn't label the vulva. Almost a third said they wouldn't feel comfortable talking about gynaecological symptoms with a doctor or showing their vagina to one. The survey was done for the Eve Appeal, which commented: 'This combination of ignorance and embarrassment could be costing lives.'

Just like with delays in endo diagnoses, a fair portion of the delays in diagnoses for gynaecological cancers—womb/uterine cancer, ovarian cancer, cervical cancer, vulval cancer, vaginal cancer—are caused by women not reporting symptoms to their doctors. Athena Lamnisos, the chief executive officer of the Eve Appeal, told me that euphemisms used by women when reporting gynaecological symptoms are sometimes so obscure that doctors don't know what they're talking about. One doctor believed, until almost the end of a ten-minute consultation, that a patient was talking about her bladder when she was actually trying to report gynaecological problems.

Research also shows that doctors often dismiss general symptoms such as bloating or irregular bleeding, or they attribute bloating to gastrointestinal issues. But when women are able to say with certainty what's normal and what's unusual for them, doctors gain a clearer picture and diagnosis can happen faster.

Half the world has these parts—there's nothing shameful or dirty about them. Imagine if we all started talking about our menstrual cycles, vaginas and vulvas more: we'd understand ourselves a bit better and get treatment faster, potentially saving lives.

Here's a correctly labelled diagram:

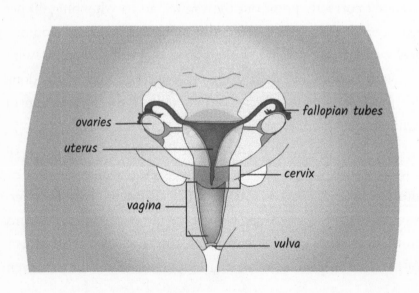

OVARIES

The ovaries are gonads, which are the primary reproductive organs. The male version is the testicles—the balls. Gonads have two jobs: to produce sex hormones and sex cells.

Women and other people with female sex organs generally each have two ovaries. About the size and shape of almonds—tiny considering how much work they do!—they get larger during the reproductive years and shrink again after menopause. They're situated on either side of the uterus (a.k.a. the womb), attached by thin ligaments.

People with female sex organs are typically born with all the sex cells we'll ever produce, while those with male sex organs continue to produce new sperm throughout their lives, although the amount and quality of sperm decreases with age.

The female sex cells are called eggs, or oocytes. At 20 weeks' gestation—about halfway through our development as a foetus—our bodies are storing about seven million follicles that contain immature eggs. By the time we're born, that number will be down to about two million follicles (and unmatured eggs) stored in our ovaries, waiting to be developed and released. When we start having a period we have about 400,000 eggs left. So where do they all go?

Well, the eggs we're born with aren't yet mature. Each month our ovaries develop the eggs we're born with into mature eggs ready to participate in the fertilisation process with sperm—but the ovaries don't just choose one egg to develop at a time. Initially, all eggs are surrounded by a sac called a follicle, basically a single layer of cells. During every cycle, cells will divide—so one cell becomes two, then they become four and so on—as the egg within it matures and

23

follicles grow progressively bigger. Some follicles can't cope with this rapid development and die off.

Eventually, one follicle dominates and a mature egg is released by one ovary each month—this is what happens when we ovulate. Just as thousands of sperm compete to merge with an egg as it travels along the fallopian tubes, a battle of eggs takes place within the ovaries to produce the fittest possible one for release. From the time we're born our ovaries do this each month, but until we're menstruating they don't receive a hormonal signal from the brain telling them to release an egg, so those follicles and eggs just die. Think of it as a dress rehearsal: they're getting ready for puberty and reproduction.

Producing oocytes, eggs or sex cells is the first job of the ovaries. Their second job is to produce sex hormones. In women and other people with female reproductive organs, the main sex hormones are oestrogen and progesterone but they also produce a small amount of testosterone.

Oestrogen is produced by everyone but is more important for women. The oestrogen produced in the ovaries is called oestradiol, and its main aim is to look after the female reproductive system, including the organs and other sex characteristics such as the uterus, vagina, breasts, hips and pelvis.

Progesterone, which means 'for pregnancy', prepares the lining of the womb for implantation, produces nutrients for an early embryo and prepares a mother's breasts for milk production during pregnancy. It also influences levels of sexual desire.

Both oestrogen and progesterone play an important part in the menstrual cycle. I'll cover that a bit more in the next chapter.

FALLOPIAN TUBES

The fallopian tubes connect the ovaries to the uterus and have three main functions: to carry an egg from the ovary to the uterus, to transport sperm to an egg, and to provide a good environment for fertilisation.

Each fallopian tube is connected to an upper corner of the uterus and reaches out, but isn't directly attached to, an ovary. The tubes are narrow ducts of 10 to 13 centimetres in length and 0.5 to 1.2 centimetres in diameter. The end of each tube closest to the ovary has an outer layer of fibres called fimbriae that reach out just over the ovary, which sits below them. During ovulation, the fimbriae contract close to the ovary's surface in order to guide the released egg into the fallopian tubes.

The channel of a fallopian tube is lined with a mucous membrane producing secretions that help keep sperm and eggs alive. This membrane contains tiny hairlike structures called cilia and is surrounded by three layers of muscle tissue. This muscle contracts, producing waves that work with the cilia to move an egg or sperm along the fallopian tubes.

If pregnancy occurs, the magic happens in a fallopian tube: that's where the male sperm and female egg combine to form a zygote. Whether the egg is fertilised or not, it takes three to four days to travel along the fallopian tube and enter the uterus.

UTERUS (WOMB)

A hollow organ, the uterus is about the size and shape of an upside-down pear. It sits inside a woman's pelvic cavity between the bladder and rectum. It's more commonly called the womb and, as you probably know—since this is the part most of us get taught at school—it's the organ where human beings grow before birth.

The uterus is 6 to 8 centimetres long. Its width varies—at the top, where the fallopian tubes attach on each side, it's about 6 centimetres wide: picture the base of the pear. The bottom end is about half this width and forms the cervix.

It's helpful to think of the uterus as a balloon. When it doesn't contain a foetus, its sides stick together. Once an embryo is implanted and a woman is pregnant, the uterus expands and hollows out to make room for the foetus to grow.

The inside lining, the endometrium, is a mucous membrane that changes in thickness throughout the menstrual cycle. The main goal of the endometrium is to nourish an embryo and foetus. The endometrium also produces fluid that helps to keep sperm and eggs alive.

The uterine wall is made up of three layers of muscle that are flexible and incredibly strong, allowing the uterus to greatly expand while the foetus grows. Then, during childbirth, this muscle contracts to push the baby out through the cervix and into the world down the vaginal canal. It also contracts to expel the endometrium during menstruation—and this is what some women feel when they have period pain.

The weaker sex? The uterus would beg to differ.

CERVIX

A thin passage about 2 to 3 centimetres long, the cervix opens out into the body of the uterus at one end. At the other, where it connects to the vagina, it contains a small hole that opens and closes during the menstrual cycle. If you have female sex organs and you're in a private place, stick your middle finger up your vagina, and at the very top you should feel a soft piece of slimy flesh of a similar shape to the tip of a nose; this is the tip of your cervix, known as the external os. The hole opens to allow menstrual blood to flow out. The cervix is really hard to see, and imagine, but the Beautiful Cervix Project has solved that problem with its collection of gorgeous (in my opinion!) photographs of cervixes that show the changes in shape and mucus throughout the cycle. You can visit the website beautifulcervix.com to see for yourself.

Think of the cervix as a security guard. It wants to protect the uterus from germs, so it keeps a tight hold on the door for the most part. But it does have to let sperm in and mucus (known as discharge), menstrual blood, babies and placentas out.

At the vagina end of the cervix is a sphincter muscle: ring-shaped, these muscles expand and contract to let fluids in and out of an opening. (Another effective sphincter muscle is the anus.) Like the uterine wall, the cervix is strong and flexible—it opens a little during ovulation and menstruation, and opens a lot during childbirth, growing to about 10 centimetres in diameter. Ever heard the phrase—maybe on *One Born Every Minute*—'She's 10 centimetres dilated'? That means the cervix has fully opened and a mother should get ready to push! Needless to say, this is pretty painful.

If you've ever worried about a tampon, menstrual cup (or something even more embarrassing) entering your uterus, there's no need—the cervix won't let it through. That goes for the penis too—it can't get past the cervix to enter a uterus, so forget any old wives' tales, urban myths or any other story you've heard to the contrary. This small but vital part of the

27

body is an excellent firewall. But you can get things stuck in your vagina behind your cervix, so it's always best to be careful with inserting objects and see a doctor immediately if something does get jammed up there.[2]

The cervix is more than a passageway: it also produces discharge as an extra barrier to germs and unwanted guests. Its inner lining produces a thick mucus that fills the passageway to prevent anything flowing between the uterus and vagina. During ovulation, the mucus thins in order to allow sperm into the uterus. This is why discharge looks different at ovulation—it has a sticky, almost egg-white consistency. When you see it on your knickers, that can be a sign you're fertile.

During pregnancy, the mucus thickens to stop germs getting to the foetus. Pregnant women often notice this discharge on their knickers too—it's totally normal.

VAGINA

The word 'vagina' is a stunning reminder of everything wrong with Western society when it comes to women's bodies. How did I get through thirteen years of education believing my vagina was my external genitalia? I'd feel stupid admitting this, only study after study shows I'm not alone. I don't remember the exact moment I realised my vagina was not, in fact, my external genitalia but the muscular tube that leads from the vulva—the umbrella term for the external genitalia—to the cervix, but it was some time during university days. Even then, I persisted for a while. At the time I didn't know any other terms used to describe it, at least not in high rotation.

To be perfectly honest, I'd grown up calling it my front bottom. Only when a boyfriend laughed uncontrollably at the term did I realise how ridiculous it sounded. I was raised Catholic; my family wasn't pious or strictly religious—we didn't go to mass every weekend, and my parents divorced in my teenage years, but I was sent to Catholic primary and secondary schools. My mum had been raised in a strict Catholic family, and although she was an open-minded, liberal woman who talked to us about puberty, sex and love, it's incredible how Catholic guilt lingers.

I mean, front bottom. Really?

I'd still be laughing if I hadn't worked out the purpose of these whitewashing names. What could better erase curiosity and impede exploration than calling a girl's genitals her front bottom? Thanks to the internet and an explosion of female-friendly news outlets, the words 'vulva' and 'labia' have become more well known. However, Eve Appeal CEO Athena Lamnisos tells me these words are still mostly unsayable. She knows better than most the consequences of this ignorance. 'Only one in seven women can name one of the gynaecological cancers, let alone five,' she tells me. 'And there's woeful lack of awareness around signs and symptoms. That's for a whole variety of reasons, but where embarrassment and stigma and taboo intersect are very much part of it. It's very different for men's reproductive organs, they can look down and across the urinal and see their reproductive organs on a daily basis—whereas women, it's either between our legs or in our pelvises, so it's literally a mystery to many women as to what their bodies, certainly what their vulvas, actually look like.'

Lamnisos recounts difficulties with signing up ambassadors. One well-meaning high-profile celebrity agreed to the role but reneged when the Appeal told them that they'd have to use the correct anatomical words 'vulva', 'vagina' and 'labia' in public—it was too big an ask. Television producers still baulk when Lamnisos says 'bleeding' on a live show and have told her to consider viewers who might be eating dinner.

Why are the natural functions of the female body still considered so vulgar? We'll get to that later.

For now, let's return to our vaginas. This muscular tube is about 9 centimetres long and, like the uterus, it's folded shut unless penetrated; this keeps it waterproof and helps prevent germs getting in. It acts as the birth canal to carry the baby from the uterus. As an added layer of protection, your two labia majora (we'll get to this soon) partly cover the vaginal opening. Amazingly, the vagina stretches both in length and width during sex and childbirth, and it shrinks after menopause. Menstrual blood and discharge also flow from the cervix through the vagina.

The inner lining of the vagina varies in thickness throughout life and the menstrual cycle, and it responds to hormones. It's thickest and most elastic during ovulation, when the body is trying its hardest to get a sperm and egg to meet and fertilise. At the same time, rising levels of oestrogen gradually increase secretions in the vagina, lubricating it—the vagina doesn't produce mucus but is covered in fluid that seeps in through its walls. The surface of the lining is acidic, which protects against germs.

By the way, this is a very good reason never to have a vaginal facial or vaginal steam. Don't believe anyone who recommends products to make the vagina healthier or smell better, unless they're a qualified medical practitioner. The vagina's pH level is sensitive, so 'cleaning' it could actually make it more prone to infections and bad smells. A bad-smelling vagina is a sign that something's wrong, and a health professional is the only person who should be consulted about this.

The vagina is always moist but it becomes more lubricated when a woman is aroused, making penetration by a penis, sex toy or fingers easier and more pleasurable. Some of the wetness comes from glands in the cervix, along with the two Bartholin's glands behind each side of the vaginal opening. However, arousal and lubrication don't always perfectly correlate—and I'll tell you more about that in Chapter 4. It should really go without saying that each of us should be intimately acquainted with our genitals, whether or not this involves sexual stimulation. If you notice a lump or any other abnormalities, you should speak to your doctor immediately.

VULVA

The vulva is the umbrella term for every part of the female external genitalia. It's what I used to refer to as the vagina, and many millions of other women still do. The vulva is called a lot of other things: front bottom (ahem), pussy, cunt, fanny, fandango (another name we used as kids), vag, minge, bearded clam, moist centre, vajayjay, twat, muff, lady garden, noo noo, tuppence, downstairs and many more names besides. Every culture has its pet terms for the vulva, and is there anything wrong with that, really?

Well, it depends. If you use a pet name as a general reference but are aware of the correct terms, then it's no big deal. But we should ask ourselves, what's the point of a pet term and the context in which it's being used? Is the pet name being used because there's shame involved in using the anatomical one?

Is it specific or does it lump a whole group of body parts into one to create confusion rather than clarity? Words matter because they aid understanding and allow us to express what we like, don't like, what's normal for us and what feels new, wrong, different, wonderful or disturbing. If we think the whole vulva is our vagina, how do we report a lump on our labia? If we don't touch ourselves occasionally, how do we know there are different parts that feel and act differently?

I'm not expecting everyone to dump their pet names immediately—after all, we're hardly going to urge our partner in the heat of the moment to stroke our labia minora! But I'd like to think we can all learn the correct terms and not be embarrassed to use them when appropriate, especially when it comes to our health.

So, what do we actually mean when we use the term 'vulva'? Well, it's what we see when we look between our legs with a mirror. At the front, the small mound of fatty tissue that protects the pubic bone and becomes covered with hair during puberty is called the mons pubis or the mound of Venus. This fatty tissue splits and parts between our legs to become the labia majora; that's the outer part of what some people call the flaps or lips. On the inside of the labia majora are another set of lips, the labia minora. The clitoral hood—the piece of skin covering the clitoral glans—is located at the front tip, where the labia meet, while the vestibulum is right in the middle.

The most important thing to understand about the vulva is that just like the human face, no two will be identical. They come in so many shapes, sizes and colours that it's hard to say what's normal—all you really have to know is what's normal

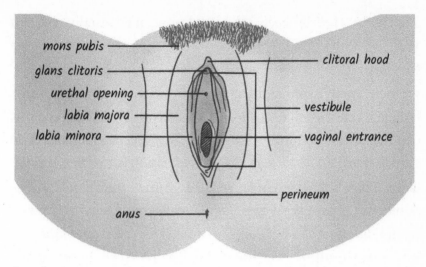

The vulva

for you. Unfortunately, we live in a world where most of the vulvas in popular culture have been censored, airbrushed to exclude details or surgically altered.

Perhaps the growth in rates of labiaplasty (cosmetic surgery on the vulva) is partly a result of people not seeing enough variety of vulvas and being led to believe what we see in porn is normal for everyone. Often labiaplasty is performed to make the inner labia shorter than the outer, but protruding inner labia are common and totally normal. According to research published in *BMJ Open* in 2016, labiaplasty increased threefold in Australia between 2003 and 2013.[3] Researchers surveyed 443 GPs and found that 54 per cent had been asked about labiaplasty; of those, 35 per cent of the requests came from girls under the age of eighteen, when labia haven't even finished developing.

One of the most gratifying pieces of art I've ever seen is a wall of labia in the Museum of Old and New Art in Tasmania.

The Great Wall of Vagina (yes, I know, it's actually a Great Wall of Vulvas, sigh) was created by the UK artist Jamie McCartney, who took a plaster cast of the genitals of 400 women aged from eighteen to 76. This great wall shows female anatomy in all its wonderful diversity. More recently, the British photographer Laura Dodsworth has embarked on a project called *Womanhood: The bare reality* in which she has taken photos of the vulvas of 100 women and gender non-conforming people. When *The Guardian* published an extract from Dodsworth's book, accompanied by a selection of images, under the headline 'Me and my vulva: 100 women reveal all', a man helpfully explained on Twitter: 'The correct word is vagina.'[4] Sigh again. This art should be in every sex education textbook in the world.

LABIA MAJORA AND LABIA MINORA

The labia majora—also called the outer labia or outer lips—along with the labia minora—inner labia or inner lips—protect the sensitive interior parts of the vulva, particularly the vaginal opening and the urethra. The labia majora's outside walls are covered with regular skin and grow pubic hair. It's made of a fatty tissue to protect the inner vulva but, as I said above, that doesn't mean it's bigger, thicker or longer than the labia minora—just like some people's second toe is longer than their big toe, some people's labia majora will be smaller than their labia minora.

The labia minora aren't covered in skin: they're mucous membranes full of nerve endings, so they can be sensitive and pleasurable to touch. When blood rushes to the genitals during arousal, the labia minora swell up, becoming engorged.

What many of us are not taught at school is how the vulva changes during puberty. We all know this is when people grow pubic hair for the first time, but that's not the only change that takes place in female genitals. During puberty, the labia minora grows. Some teenagers may never have noticed these inner lips before, and suddenly they're hanging down longer than the outer lips. If people aren't taught this is a normal part of puberty, and the only images of vulvas they're exposed to are airbrushed, is it any wonder they worry about how they look and want to change it? But just like breasts grow and hips start to take shape during puberty, labia also grow and change shape.

VESTIBULUM

Just like a vestibule in a building, the vestibulum is the area between the entrance and the interior. If you pull the labia apart and look at the space between them, you'll see two holes. The tiny hole at the front is the urethra, where your urine comes out; the bigger hole behind that, closer to the anus, is the vaginal opening.

A lot of people are confused about these holes—and, in fact, many don't even know there are two. Because a single hole in the tip of the penis expels both urine and sperm, people assume that female anatomy also has only one hole. But penises aren't equipped with a birth canal or a passageway to expel menstrual blood: the urethra is too small for those jobs, so people with female sex organs need two holes.

One hot Sydney summer's day when I was about thirteen, my friend and I wanted another friend to come swimming with us. She told us she couldn't because she had her period, so we decided it was time she started using tampons like we did. We said we'd coach her from outside the bathroom door. When she repeatedly said, 'The hole's not big enough', it dawned on us that she didn't know she had two holes—three, if we include the anus.

You can imagine my surprise when I was watching the second season of *Orange is the New Black* and came across an episode devoted to pointing out that there are two holes in the vestibulum. Apparently this ignorance is so widespread that a popular TV show made an episode about it. How can this be? Half the world has this anatomy! In that episode, a transwoman, Sophia—played by the brilliant Laverne Cox—explains female anatomy to the other women in prison, and soon enough the newly educated inmates are fighting over a mirror to check it all out. To butcher the words of Sophia, for the love of God, girls, get a mirror and get to know what your vulva looks like!

CLITORIS

Now we get to my favourite part of the body: the most sensitive organ humans possess. But it's a sadly ignored, misunderstood and undervalued organ. There are 8000 nerve endings in the tip of the clitoris alone—that's more than anywhere else in the human body and twice the number of those in a penis. The clitoris is made up of a mixture of erectile tissue, muscle and nerves, and can swell as much as 300 per cent when engorged.

A lot people think the clitoris begins and ends at the glans clitoris—but that's only the external part. You may have heard the clitoris described as the size and shape of a raisin or pea; even the *Oxford English Dictionary* still defines it as 'A small, sensitive, erectile part of the female genitals at the anterior end

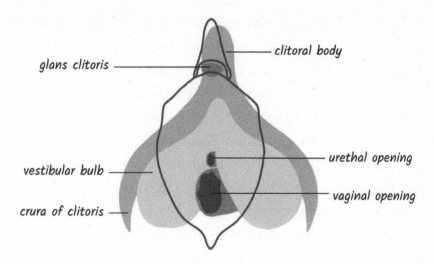

glans clitoris

clitoral body

urethal opening

vestibular bulb

vaginal opening

crura of clitoris

A clitoris, most of which is internal

of the vulva.' Although this isn't the full picture, even today many official textbooks have got it wrong.

The full internal and external clitoris is the shape of a wishbone with dangly earrings or bulbs between the outer legs. The glans clitoris connects to a body or shaft of the internal clitoris. Its two leg-like structures—the crura—wrap tightly around the vaginal wall when aroused and erect, and its two bulb-like structures—the vestibular bulbs—sit underneath the labia and also become erect when aroused. The whole structure is attached to the pubic bone via ligaments.

Because of its internal structure, the clitoris can be stimulated via the vagina, urethra and anus, as well as, of course, through external stimulation of the labia and glans clitoris. In other words, all female orgasms are clitoral orgasms.

As far back as the 1840s, a German anatomist by the name of Georg Ludwig Kobelt described the organ's internal structure, including the fact it's composed of erectile tissue similar to the penis. But it seems this knowledge was forgotten for many years—one 1940s version of the medical bible *Gray's Anatomy* even left out the clitoris altogether. Hmmm.

It took a female doctor, Australian urologist Professor Helen O'Connell, to rewrite the medical textbooks on female anatomy[5] with her groundbreaking work on the clitoris. In 1998, she published a scientific paper showing conclusively that the glans clitoris was only the tip of the iceberg of the organ itself. Her work mapped the key nerves, blood vessels and connective tissue, allowing surgeons to better protect loss of sexual function in female pelvic surgery—something not done until then.

O'Connell was motivated to uncover the truth about the clitoris by the textbooks she was forced to study in medical school, which showed the clitoris as only the glans. She dissected cadavers, and later conducted MRI scans to show the full body of the clitoris and its rich blood flow and nerve pathways.

Her work was followed by two French scientists (one of whom became famous for reconstructing the clitorises of female genital mutilation victims) who in 2009 created the first 3-D model of the full clitoris structure. Only then did non-medical people gain a complete understanding of what the clitoris looked like—2009!

Stunned by the widespread lack of knowledge about the clitoris, in 2017 Australian artist Alli Sebastian Wolf created a human-size (100:1 scale) anatomically correct model of the clitoris covered in glitter: the *Glitoris*. It even shows the eighteen different interconnected parts of muscle, nerves and erectile tissue beneath the surface. Sebastian Wolf says it's 'a playful way to educate and celebrate this misunderstood organ'.[6] Her *Glitoris* is now world-renowned—it has appeared on stage with the musician Amanda Palmer and in the pages of *The Guardian*, and it travels widely for performances, talks and education sessions with a performance group, the Clitorati, who call themselves 'ambassadors for the clit'.[7]

HYMEN

The hymen is perhaps the most inconsequential part of the female reproductive system biologically, and the most consequential socially.

Before we get into what it is, let's deal with what it isn't: a sign of virginity. The hymen myth is one of the most dangerous in existence. The simple fact is, the only way to tell if someone is a virgin is to ask them and believe the answer.

The hymen is a thin membrane that sits 1 to 2 centimetres inside the vaginal opening. Just like the labia and many other human features, hymens come in all shapes and sizes, and change during puberty. It's a mistake to think of the hymen as a seal that covers the vaginal opening completely and has to be broken at some stage. In most cases, the hymen is a bit like a doughnut, with a crescent-shaped hole in the middle that allows people with a vagina to menstruate, use tampons and masturbate without even noticing its existence. In rare cases—about 2 per cent—the membrane does cover the vaginal opening. This might not be noticed until menstruation when the blood can't get out, causing a lot of pain; fortunately it can be fixed with a minor surgical procedure. The procedure might also be necessary for hymens that have a very small hole in the middle, or cover the vaginal opening with multiple small holes like a sieve. For some people, the hymen is barely visible and wears away completely as we grow up.

The hymen is elastic but not as elastic as the vaginal wall, and it's at the narrowest point of the vagina, so many activities can stretch and tear it. Sexual penetration is one, using tampons is another, along with bike riding, horseriding, gymnastics and other exercise. This can cause bleeding and pain, but it can heal itself with no scar.[8] Since the hymen has no use in women—in the same way that men have no use for nipples—it doesn't matter at what stage in life this happens.

But the hymen is so important culturally that clinics around the world offer hymen-repair surgery so women bleed during vaginal sex on their wedding night—regardless of the original shape of their hymen. Not every person with a vagina bleeds the first time they have sex. Keep in mind that even without breaking a hymen, the vaginal wall can bleed during rough sex or if there isn't enough lubrication. Some cultures display

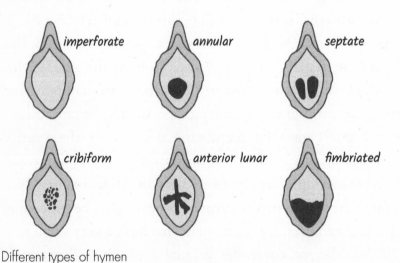

Different types of hymen

bloody bedsheets after a husband and wife's first night together as proof of the wife's virginity, and this act is the cause of much pain and suffering.

Female virginity is a social construct used to keep women submissive to men. What does virginity mean, anyway? When I was at school there was talk of girls having anal sex so they'd stay a virgin—how ludicrous! I was a teenager during the Bill Clinton–Monica Lewinsky affair when Clinton famously said he 'did not have sexual relations with that woman, Ms Lewinsky'. When it came out they'd engaged in oral sex, a major debate took place in the mainstream media about what constituted 'sex'. Is oral sex 'sex'? How can vaginal penetration by a penis be the only form of sex? Are gay people virgins forever? A major reason these delineations are seen as important is that female virginity is highly valued and controlled. I'll talk more about sexuality in Chapter 4 but for now, the most important point to understand is that the hymen has nothing to do with virginity.

———

So that's our reproductive system. Unfortunately, these aren't the only misconceptions bedevilling our understanding of women's health.

CHAPTER 2

'Worse than the Loch Ness monster': menstruation and menopause

The myths and taboos around menstruation are of biblical proportions. Take this from Leviticus, the third book of the Old Testament and Torah: 'If a woman have an issue, and her issue in her flesh be blood, she shall be put apart seven days: and whosoever toucheth her shall be unclean until the even' (Leviticus 15:19).

Strong myths around cleanliness for centuries have prevented menstruating women from preparing food, having sex, visiting places of religious worship and even entering the home. These myths are often fortified by social taboos that prevent women from talking about their menstrual cycles, and cultural prescriptions about which menstrual hygiene products are acceptable for women to use. In India, for example, in some states it was believed a woman would go blind or never get married if she used sanitary pads; instead, rural women used leaves, ash, sawdust and old rags—which they couldn't dry in the sun so were never disinfected.[1] A lack of access to any kind of menstrual hygiene products or private toilet facilities still prevents millions of girls around the world from attending school each month. This isn't just bad for their education, limiting their life opportunities, it's also bad for their health: in India, 70 per cent of all reproductive illnesses are caused by poor menstrual hygiene.[2] It can also affect maternal mortality.

And if you think this isn't a problem in the Western world, consider the Australian Aboriginal woman who was fined $500 for stealing a $6.75 packet of tampons from an outback service station. She said she stole them for someone else who was 'too ashamed' to buy them herself.[3]

Meanwhile, UK food banks have reported an increase in demand for sanitary products, with reports of people using toilet paper and staying at home during their periods, or stuffing socks and newspaper in their underwear. The problem is so large-scale that Scotland piloted a free sanitary products scheme in 2018, which it expanded in 2019.[4]

In June 2018, Labour MP Danielle Rowley stood up in the British House of Commons to announce she had her period and it has cost her £25 (A$45) that week already. 'You know the average cost of a period in the UK over a year is £500. Many women can't afford this. What is the minister doing to address period poverty?' she asked. Back in 2000, the UK Labour government had reduced the sales tax (VAT) on sanitary products from 17.5 to 5 per cent but said it couldn't reduce it any further under European Union rules. In response to Rowley, the minister for women, Victoria Atkins, promised to remove sales tax on menstrual products once the UK's exit from the EU was final, and said her government was 'watching with interest' the Scottish government's program to deliver free products to those in need.[5]

In October 2018, Australia finally caught up with much of the US in dropping the sales tax on menstrual hygiene products. We've seen how lack of access to menstrual products holds girls back from school and women from work; we know lack of access to hygienic products causes disease and illness. Yet for two decades the Australian government refused to lift the sales tax on these products despite the loud demands of feminists. While a policy to lift the tax was briefly flirted with in 2015, the government later reneged, as did the Opposition Labor Party, which claimed it 'couldn't afford to lose the revenue'.[6] Women earn 17.9 per cent less than men in Australia. Women do the bulk of unpaid labour, such as cooking, cleaning and housework, with Australian women being among the most overworked in the world. Australian women retire with 53 per cent of the superannuation that men retire with and are significantly more likely to experience poverty than men. And the government needs more revenue from us?

As New York governor Andrew Cuomo noted upon repealing the state sales tax on menstruation products in 2016, removing these taxes is a 'matter of social and economic justice'.[7]

But it's not only cost and access holding women back. In almost every country, myths around menstruation continue to prosper and a tampon falling out of a handbag remains a sadly embarrassing event. The period-tracking app, Clue, compiled a list of 36 superstitions about periods from around the world: avoiding cooking, washing hair, having sex, swimming or taking a bath are common superstitions across cultures and continents. Tom Rankin, a program manager supporting water, sanitation and hygiene projects for the human rights agency Plan International Australia, told me that in parts of eastern Africa, menstruating women aren't allowed to cook or fetch water: 'There's all these myths, like if you milk a cow, the cow will go dry. Or if you tend a garden, the garden will be unproductive. Or if you walk over water pipes, it contaminates the water,' he said. 'All these . . . myths that relate to menstruation create these enormous social barriers for women and girls just to participate freely in society.'

Medical science has played a historic role in perpetuating ideas that menstruation is unsafe, unclean and unmentionable. We'll see in the next chapter, on hysteria, how women's reproductive functions have been pathologised and suspected throughout history, and used to justify women's limited role in society. Dr Kate Young, a public health researcher at Monash University, has highlighted how even today medicine 'endorses menstruation as a leakage that transgresses bodily boundaries, supposedly evidencing women's inherent lack of control over their bodies and reinforcing their "need" to remain in the private sphere'.[8]

Such myths thrive in a culture of silence, where whispers that enforce unscientific practices go unchallenged because the taboo of talking about menstruation reigns supreme over education and facts. In the US, an ad was banned from the New York subway because 'of the nature of the language used'. 'Underwear for women with periods', was the offending sentence. As Deirdre Hynds noted in the *Irish Times*,[9] at the time the ad was banned in 2015 the city's Metropolitan Transportation Authority had seen fit to approve ads for 'breast augmentation' and a photo of a woman being choked with a necktie in an ad for a *Fifty Shades of Grey* film.

Making talk of periods shameful is a key strategy in the oppression of women worldwide—and it happens in every modern society. But the menstrual cycle, and changes to it, are signs of so much regarding the health of everyone who menstruates.

The American actress Courteney Cox was the first person to say 'period' on television—that was in 1985 in a Tampax commercial, and it hasn't been said much since. In its work with girls around the world, Plan International has found that menstruation must be discussed at a community level if stigmas are to be broken down. The greatest success is seen when men and boys become actively involved in the conversation, because men are often the enforcers of social stigmas and cultural norms. This isn't so different in the Western world, which is why campaigners in Australia, New Zealand and the United Kingdom have all told me how imperative it is to teach boys about all aspects of menstruation—including what's a normal amount of period pain—in schools. Only when menstruation stops being secret women's business will life improve for everyone who struggles to enjoy full dignity and social inclusion when they have their period. Some health campaigners want menstruation to be taught in health lessons, separate from sex education, because of the shame and stigma involved when it comes to sex. Indeed, separating health from sex and gender issues remains a massive hurdle to overcome.

Our menstrual cycle can be a key clue to our health, so noticing when things change is important, as is being able to confidently talk about our cycle to healthcare professionals. Knowing the facts is also the single biggest threat to the survival of dangerous and repressive myths.

We need to know what's normal as opposed to what's common. Period pain is common; period pain that interferes with daily life isn't normal and should be investigated. Bleeding between periods is common, but it isn't necessarily normal and should be reported to a doctor. The Eve Appeal found that almost 20 per cent of women wouldn't report abnormal bleeding to a doctor—a disturbingly high figure, and one that needs to change. A strong social conditioning in people who menstruate makes us not want to be 'difficult', and maybe some don't know if abnormal bleeding is a cause for concern.

We must destroy the taboo on talking about periods. It's not only education that needs to change, it's conversation.

But first: facts.

THIS IS HOW YOUR MENSTRUAL CYCLE WORKS

From puberty to menopause, menstrual cycles begin and end on the first day of the period. Cycle lengths vary from woman to woman, and from culture to culture. For most Western women, the average cycle is about 28 days but anything from 23 to 35 days is normal. Most fluctuate slightly from cycle to cycle and throughout reproductive life, though some lucky ducks have a stickler cycle that turns up on the same day each time. If only! Mine ranges from 24 to 35 days, and I never know which I'm gonna get.

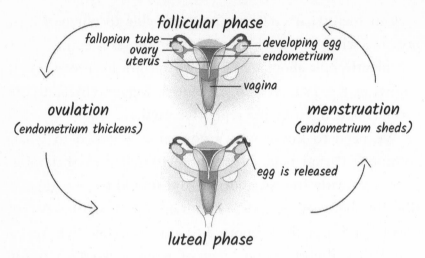

follicular phase

fallopian tube
ovary
uterus

developing egg
endometrium

vagina

ovulation
(endometrium thickens)

menstruation
(endometrium sheds)

egg is released

luteal phase

The menstrual cycle

The menstrual cycle is divided into two phases: the follicular (the first) and the luteal (the second). The follicular phase varies in length but the luteal phase is almost always 14 days long. So, if a cycle is 28 days long, the follicular phase will be 14 days and the luteal phase will be 14 days. If a cycle is 35 days long, the follicular phase will be 21 days and the luteal phase will be 14 days. If the cycle is 23 days long, the follicular phase will be nine days and the luteal phase will be 14 days. There are some exceptions, but even then the length of the luteal phase won't change throughout the reproductive years.

The follicular phase

Day one of the follicular phase is when bleeding begins.

Remember follicles? They're the cellular sacs in which eggs wait to mature. During the first phase of the menstrual cycle these follicles develop, preparing multiple eggs for ovulation.

Throughout the follicular phase, oestrogen is the dominant

hormone. On day one, when the uterus is busy getting rid of the lining it doesn't need (no egg has been fertilised), both oestrogen and progesterone levels are low. This alerts the pituitary gland in the brain—part of the hypothalamic–pituitary–ovarian axis—to start producing something called follicle-stimulating hormone to . . . you guessed it, stimulate the follicles to start maturing those eggs.

At around day seven, if you have an internal ultrasound you can usually start to see a number of follicles developing in each ovary. They could be up to 6 to 7 millimetres at this stage. As they grow the follicles produce oestrogen, and the bigger they get the more oestrogen they produce; this causes the uterine lining to grow in preparation for the implantation of a fertilised egg. Over a number of days, one follicle will usually become dominant. When it reaches around 18 to 20 millimetres in diameter, oestrogen levels are so high that it sends a signal to the pituitary gland to produce luteinising hormone, which activates the egg so it's ready for the fertilisation process, then releases it from the ovary.

This point marks ovulation, and the beginning of second phase of the menstrual cycle.

The luteal phase

In the second phase of the menstrual cycle, the egg goes in search of a partner in the form of sperm.

Once released, the egg survives for a maximum of 24 hours. Hard to believe, isn't it? All that hard work developing, it wins the battle of the ovum, then it only lives for a day! But textbooks have wrongly presented sperm as the go-getting gamete that hunts down and pierces the waiting egg. As Emily Martin laid bare in her 1991 paper, 'The egg and the sperm: How science has constructed a romance based on stereotypical male-female roles',[10] the egg is far from passive. Martin found that even though several biologists have confirmed the egg plays an active role in attracting and capturing semen—while semen is quite weak and slippery, incapable of implanting without the egg's participation—textbooks and other learning materials have continued to use language that centres the sperm as active and the egg as passive. 'The imagery keeps alive some of the hoariest old stereotypes about damsels in distress and their strong male rescuers,' wrote Martin. 'That these stereotypes are now being written in at the level of the cell constitutes a powerful move to make them seem so natural as to be beyond alteration.'

Once released the egg goes in search of sperm, which has often been bumbling around the fallopian tubes for hours or even days. As the eager egg bobs along the tube and the sperm wait, progesterone takes charge. When a follicle releases an egg, it breaks down and becomes the corpus luteum, which produces progesterone. In the follicular phase, oestrogen helped build up the endometrium in the uterus; now, progesterone takes the lead role in maintaining it to make sure it's a welcoming environment for a fertilised egg. While progesterone is on the rise, it prevents the uterus from contracting to expel the endometrium. It also tells the pituitary gland not to produce follicle-stimulating and luteinising hormones so that new eggs aren't developing while our activated egg is on the prowl for a partner.

If the egg isn't fertilised, the corpus luteum dies out and stops producing progesterone. With progesterone levels plummeting, the endometrium stops thickening, and the uterus can contract and expel its lining. The pituitary gland can now produce its hormones again, so follicles begin to develop and the cycle restarts.

PREGNANCY

If a fertilised egg implants in the endometrium, a hormone called human chorionic gonadotropin is produced. This tells the corpus luteum to keep producing progesterone, along with a type of oestrogen; the progesterone prevents menstruation and continues to make sure the endometrium is a nourishing environment for an embryo. The corpus luteum maintains this role until about week eight of pregnancy, when the placenta takes over and the corpus luteum dies out. So the human chorionic gonadotropin determines whether the corpus luteum lives or dies, and therefore whether you menstruate—that's why this is the hormone that pregnancy tests look for.

Something happens to a lot of people when they start trying to become pregnant. Many of us have spent a good portion of our adult lives stressing about accessing the morning-after pill, waiting anxiously for our periods to arrive, and worrying about broken condoms, missed pills, a bout of vomiting or diarrhoea—and then one day, all this is turned on its head and we start dreading our periods. We're back to playing close attention to our cycles but for the opposite reasons. Then we discover that an egg only lives for a day, and we're like, *OHMYGOD, what the hell?! How many times did I needlessly get the morning-after pill? How many months did I waste worrying whether I was pregnant when I had sex at a time when it was next to impossible?*

Here are a few relevant facts about fertility:

- It can take sperm cells anywhere from 45 minutes to 12 hours to reach the fallopian tubes, and they can survive there for up to seven days, although normally it's about 48 hours.
- Even though millions of sperm may be ejaculated at orgasm, only a few dozen make it all the way to the fallopian tubes.
- As we saw in the previous chapter, the cervix is closed for most of the menstrual cycle, but around the time of ovulation its thick mucous plug thins to allow sperm into the uterus.

So when are you fertile?

A study of 221 healthy women looking into the timing of sexual intercourse found nearly all pregnancies resulted from intercourse in the five days before ovulation and on the day of ovulation. That would mean we're only fertile for six days per cycle.[11]

The egg and sperm fertilising in the fallopian tube doesn't equal pregnancy. There are still many, many barriers to overcome before that happens. Pregnancy only occurs when an embryo embeds in the endometrium—and this usually takes about seven days. The process fascinates me; when I was undergoing IVF, I'd stay up late into the night reading brochures and articles about it. During fertilisation, a single cell is created called a zygote, which keeps dividing into more cells roughly every 24 hours. By day five, it will have become a blastocyst, containing between 75 and 100 cells. At around day seven, the blastocyst implants in the uterine wall; this is when pregnancy begins and human chorionic gonadotropin is released.[12]

Between 30 and 70 per cent of zygotes don't make it to

implantation. Some researchers think this is because of genetic imperfections—it seems the body discards most genetically damaged fertilised cells before they become foetuses.

About 14 days after fertilisation and seven days of being snuggly embedded in the endometrium, the blastocyst becomes an embryo. This is also the stage at which most periods would usually be due. The embryo stage lasts until about week nine or ten, when it becomes a foetus.

PERIOD PAIN

Most girls, women and other people who menstruate get some amount of pain with their periods. But what is a normal amount of period pain? It's important to understand this because so many people report being told 'period pain is normal' when they complain to a medical practitioner, or even just to their friends and family.

Period pain that interferes with daily life isn't normal.

Dr Susan Evans, a gynaecologist, pain physician and chair of the Pelvic Pain Foundation of Australia, tells me, 'Normal period pain is pain on the first one to two days of bleeding that is easily managed with taking an anti-inflammatory or going on the pill.'

A number of factors could be causing period pain. One is a hormone called prostaglandins, produced by endometrial cells that form the uterine lining. When the endometrium is shed during menstruation, it releases a large amount of prostaglandins, causing the uterus to contract and expel its lining. Studies have shown that people with period pain have high levels of prostaglandins. The good news about this is that over-the-counter medicine known as nonsteroidal anti-inflammatory drugs can block the production of prostaglandins and help to ease the pain: ibuprofen (Nurofen is one of the big brands that sell this), naproxen (Naprogesic or Naprosyn) and diclofenac (Voltaren) can all be bought in most supermarkets and pharmacies, and have all been shown to work for most cases of period pain. They're more effective if taken before the pain starts or before the pain becomes severe. The Pelvic Pain Foundation of Australia has good information on how to take these drugs to manage or avoid pain.

Taking the contraceptive pill—one with more progestin (synthetic progesterone) than oestrogen—has also been proven to help manage period pain in most people, as has the Mirena intrauterine device (IUD). It's important to avoid taking opioids, like Endone or OxyContin, to treat period pain where possible, because studies show that these drugs can make chronic pain worse.

If none of these methods reduce the pain and make life easier, another issue may be at play. Endometriosis, adenomyosis, fibroids and pelvic inflammatory disease are some of the main potential causes of pain that should be investigated by a doctor at this stage. However, it may just be that you have severe period pain and no other identifiable disease. Chronic pelvic pain is now being recognised as a condition in itself that should be taken seriously. I'll talk a lot more about period pain and how it can lead to chronic pain conditions if untreated in Chapter 6. The important thing to remember here is that if period pain interferes with your daily life or happens on more than one to two days at the start of bleeding and can't be controlled with over-the-counter drugs, it's not normal and you should see a doctor.

PREMENSTRUAL SYNDROME

The neuroscience of looking at how oestrogen and progesterone influence mood is 'so new it's practically pre-pubertal',
writes the neuroscientist Dr Sarah McKay in *The Women's
Brain Book*.

Huh? Don't all women occasionally become emotional and
irrational before they get their period? Haven't some women
been acquitted of murder because of premenstrual stress?
When you really lose your shit at your loved ones, don't you
just know it must almost be that time of the month?

Well, no, yes and no. It's true that two British court cases
in the early 1980s established PMS as a defence for murder
but, as McKay notes, no study has ever shown that women's
ability to think clearly is influenced by their menstrual cycle.
And despite the best efforts of some male scientists, no one has
been able to prove that men are naturally more intelligent than
women. 'This is good news!' writes McKay. 'Our cognitive
abilities and intelligence are not held captive by hormones.'[13]

This isn't to say that PMS doesn't exist. Many women
report some physical or psychological symptoms in the days
before their period, although numbers vary widely and more
research needs to be done on this topic (surprise, surprise).
Physical symptoms commonly include tender breasts, bloating,
headaches and greasy hair or skin. Mental symptoms include
mood swings, anger, irritability, fatigue and foggy thinking.
Some women with migraines or autoimmune conditions
report their usual symptoms getting worse in the days before
menstruation.

But this syndrome has blurry edges, in that literally hundreds
of symptoms can be ascribed to it. The narrative of PMS

embedded in Western culture is based more on folklore than science. There's no widely accepted figure for the number of people who experience it, although the US Office on Women's Health says that more than 90 per cent of women will have some symptoms in the days preceding their periods, such as bloating, headaches and moodiness, while fewer than 5 per cent suffer the severe symptoms of another condition, premenstrual dysphoric disorder. Other studies claim that between 20 and 30 per cent of women suffer mild to moderate symptoms of PMS.[14]

One of the main reasons patriarchy is so successful is that it has established countless ways for women to blame ourselves for our own oppression. Girls are taught from a young age to police themselves as they try to meet society's expectations of femininity. While trying to be 'good', most women have pinned a bad mood to their menstrual cycle at one point or another. We've probably been insulted by someone who blamed PMS for the fact we're angry at them—and we may have agreed, blaming ourselves too. The idea of the menstrual cycle turning women into harridans is so entrenched in our society, as women we even buy into it ourselves. And when losing our temper happens to coincide with the premenstrual phase, we notice this and blame it on the hormones.

But this is a phenomenon called confirmation bias: we've heard about PMS our whole lives, so when we act in a way that fits the narrative, we accept it as truth.

Numerous studies have called into question the most damaging fictions about PMS: those that attribute anger and irritation to uncontrollable female hormones. Sarah Romans, a professor of psychological medicine at the University of Otago in New Zealand, has conducted two studies that show mood swings in women rarely correlate to the premenstrual phase. Her Mood in Daily Life study, which looked at nearly 80 Canadian women who kept a daily mood diary over six months, 'found little evidence to support that premenstrual phase by itself influenced mood. Instead, mood was more closely influenced by one of three culprits—lack of social support, perceived stress or poor physical health.'[15] In a separate literature review Romans conducted, she found no clear evidence of the existence of a specific premenstrual negative mood syndrome in the general population. 'This puzzlingly widespread belief needs challenging, as it perpetuates negative concepts linking female reproduction with negative emotionality,' she wrote.[16]

Jane Ussher, a professor of women's health psychology at Western Sydney University, documents in her fascinating 2006 book, *Managing the Monstrous Feminine*, that most of the psychological symptoms women put down to PMS were reactions to stresses in their lives that they silenced for the rest of the month. Across the 70 women interviewed in Australia and the UK, it was startling to observe the similarities in the causes of emotional outbursts attributed to PMS. Many spoke of the lack of support they received from their male partners, of being overwhelmed by the burden of housework and childcare, and being taken for granted by their families. Women with less of an overwhelming burden, and those who had supportive partners, tended to fare better.

In her book, Ussher speaks of the premenstrual phase as a time of vulnerability in some women, saying those who usually repress their anger or resentment at partners, children or the unfair burden of their responsibilities are more likely to let it erupt at this time. 'So the body, that old stalwart source of sin, is positioned as to blame. Don't blame men, or families, or the impossible constraints of femininity for the rage, for the frustration at lack of support or space. Blame raging hormones.'[17]

So the take-out is this: some women become more sensitive and irritable premenstrually, and a minority have a severe reaction. But this doesn't impair their ability to think or work, or make them somehow out of control—their anger is usually in response to real life stress.

Throughout history, women's reproductive organs and so-called raging hormones have been used as excuses for their exclusion from education, professional work and public space. If we are to accept that women are essentially out of control for one week in every four, then perhaps the ban on female pilots should be reinstated? Or, as Ussher suggests, what's stopping legislators from preventing women from driving cars in their premenstrual phase? (Perhaps the fact that women have fewer accidents than men, no matter what part of the cycle they're in?)

A person's lived experience should never be denied, and treatment should of course be provided for those who suffer physical or mental distress, whether or not it's cyclical. As in most areas of women's health, not enough is known about premenstrual syndrome. What is definitively known is that the normal variation in hormones throughout the menstrual cycle does *not* cause someone to be irrational, unreasonable or totally lose control.

MENOPAUSE

Just like menstruation, menopause is a natural cycle of life that's also a highly charged social construction. Both are dogged by taboos, shame, lack of education and misinformation.

There's an Amy Schumer comedy sketch in which she comes across the actors Julia Louis-Dreyfus, Tina Fey and Patricia Arquette having a picnic in the woods. They tell her they're celebrating Louis-Dreyfus's 'last fuckable day'. 'In every actress's life, the media decides when you finally reach the point where you're not believably fuckable anymore,' Louis-Dreyfus explains to Schumer.

The sketch instantly became a classic, not only because it feels so true about media and Hollywood, but also because this is how many women approach menopause. It's as though this change in their lives is the end of themselves as attractive, sexual beings. And that's because it has historically, at least in the Western world, been sold that way by some doctors and scientists.

Two seminal books helped establish this idea in Western society at a time when women were finally starting to gain some freedom. *Everything You Always Wanted to Know About Sex★ (★But Were Afraid to Ask)*, by the psychiatrist Dr David Reuben, is one of the biggest-selling books on sex of all time and later inspired a Woody Allen movie of the same name. Published in 1969, it had a profound effect on sex education and has been hailed as an integral part of the sexual revolution. It included such gems on menopausal women as: 'Having outlived their ovaries, they may have outlived their usefulness as human beings. The remaining years may be just marking time until they follow their glands into oblivion.'[18] And: 'As estrogen is shut off, a woman comes as close as she can to being a man. Increased facial hair, deepened voice, obesity, and the decline of breasts and female genitalia all contribute to a masculine appearance. Coarsened features, enlargement of the clitoris and gradual baldness complete the picture. Not really a man, but no longer a functional woman, these individuals live in a world in intersex . . . sex no longer interests them.'[19]

Sex no longer interests them? Try telling that to the women in an Australian study[20] who reported having a greater sex drive associated with a new partner following menopause. Reuben's descriptions of menopausal women are pseudoscience, better known as bullshit. When it comes to menopause, there's a lot of it around.

The American gynaecologist Dr Robert Wilson was instrumental in constructing menopause as a disease, one that could be cured by doctors with drugs. A paper he wrote with his wife, Thelma, in the *Journal of the American Geriatrics Society* in 1963 was so influential, he expanded upon it in his best-selling 1966 book, *Feminine Forever*. He was evangelical about hormone replacement therapy (HRT)—while being paid by the pharmaceutical companies that produced it—and tried to justify his position with insults: 'All post-menopausal women are castrates.' But, he urged, if women took HRT, they could be 'feminine forever'. He claimed that the benefits of HRT extended far beyond symptom relief, writing that a woman's 'breasts and genital organs will not shrivel' on the therapy: 'She will be much more pleasant to live with and will not become dull and unattractive.'[21]

It's not just medical doctors who have pushed these grotesque notions on Western women about menopause. Academic researchers have made similarly repressive claims based on questionable science. The authors of one 2013 paper claim to have discovered that women go through menopause because men of all ages prefer younger women, so older women won't be having sex and don't need to reproduce.[22]

In her book, *Inferior*, the science journalist Angela Saini does a great job documenting the raging battle among evolutionary biologists over why human females go through menopause. What emerges is clear evidence that scientists, just like people everywhere, are influenced in their collection and interpretation of data by their life experience, beliefs, and—yes—their gender.

It's important to note that the controversial paper claiming menopause exists because men don't find older women attractive, from the evolutionary biologist Rama Singh and his colleagues at McMaster University in Canada,[23] was published at a time when a growing body of evidence in evolutionary biology seemed to support the 'grandmother theory' of menopause. This theory supposes that women go through menopause because their role as grandmothers is integral in child survival, exploding myths about useless old ladies staring into oblivion and instead granting them centre stage in the survival of the human race. The American anthropologist Kristen Hawkes has spent decades collecting data to support this theory, and others have added to it. As Saini points out, when it comes to evolutionary theories on menopause, there's a trend that isn't hard to spot: 'counter-theories to the grandmother hypothesis appear to come mainly from men'.[24] Clearly, some of the men writing the science on sex and biology, and influencing how it's taught, have certain ideas about women and certain interests in maintaining the status quo.

Most women experience some unpleasant effects of menopause, but the dread women hold about this process is at least in part socially constructed. No other expected life change besides death is approached with such fear and apprehension.

Of all the myths surrounding menopause, three stand out: a woman's sex life is over, she'll gain a lot of weight and she'll turn into a maniac. None of these are certain to occur, and with knowledge and the right treatment all can be avoided or minimised. A 1992 study published in the *Psychosomatic Medicine* journal found that attitudes to menopause went some way in predicting experiences. 'Middle-aged women believe that holding negative expectations about the menopause affects the quality of the menopausal experience. Indeed, that appears to be the case, perhaps because myths can function as self-fulfilling prophecy,' wrote the study's author, K.A. Matthews.[25]

In cultures where older women are revered and granted power, they report fewer menopause symptoms than in cultures where this doesn't take place. This remains true in cultures as far apart as Rajasthan in India and in Indigenous communities in the Tiwi Islands, in northern Australia. Beverley Ayers, a psychologist from King's College London, noted this discrepancy in an article for the *Psychologist*, showing that women in India, Japan and China experience far fewer menopause symptoms than those in the West.[26]

I'm not suggesting that magical thinking will make menopause a breeze. The process of ageing presents challenges to everyone's bodies, and menopause has proven physical impacts. Sex hormones are fluctuating during this time, which can cause dramatic physical and mental effects in some women. Many of us remember how hard it was to go through puberty— facing it again, in reverse, doesn't sound like much fun.

But menopause doesn't last forever, and not all women have a terrible experience. It's not the end times—far from it. In the second season of the British sitcom *Fleabag*, a character played by Kristin Scott Thomas calls menopause 'the most wonderful fucking thing in the world'. This seems like a good time to give menopause a makeover.

As with all subjects that have been taboo, changing minds and attitudes is hard. Many brave famous women, including Jean Kittson in Australia, Jane Fonda in the USA, Kirsty Wark in the UK, and Germaine Greer, Emma Thompson, Angelina Jolie and Gillian Anderson have started to speak about their experiences of menopause, but representations of older women or of menopause itself remain rare in Western culture—at least outside of comedy, where menopausal women are usually the butt of the joke.

After the release of the French film *I Got Life!*, about a menopausal woman, the English journalist Suzanne Moore lamented the lack of representation of menopause in popular culture. 'As long as we don't have any kind of representations of menopause, in all its glory, then it will continue to be seen as a sign that a woman is somehow redundant because she can no longer reproduce. If we were to talk more openly, we would find instead that many women feel liberated, full of energy, able to take on the world, and finally free from the demands of a society that values only youth. As the heroine of this movie kicks off her shoes, dances, gardens, makes love, becomes a grandmother and hangs out with her friends, life in its messy way continues. The idea that women may indeed be less concerned about how others see them and become more of themselves is a story rarely told,' Moore wrote in *The Guardian*.[27]

Menopause cafes are popping up in workplaces all over Britain, 'where co-workers gather over cake to compare notes about the way hot sweats, aphasia (language problems), insomnia, dry vaginas and how the ins and outs of HRT might affect women's sense of wellbeing at work. Male colleagues wanting to better understand how to support their female partners are warmly welcomed,' explained Marina Benjamin, author of *The Middlepause*.[28] This development is worth applauding, and let's hope the trend kicks off around the world.

But what exactly goes on during menopause?

The biology of menopause

Understanding the biology of what causes menopause is pretty easy when you have a basic grasp of the female reproductive system. What's harder is understanding the effects, and how they relate to what's happening biologically as well as socially and psychologically during menopause.

First: what is menopause? Medically, it's when someone hasn't had a period for 12 months. Commonly, we speak of 'going through menopause' but, strictly speaking, the time leading up to the end of periods is the perimenopause. Someone isn't menopausal until 12 months since their last period. After that, they're post-menopausal.

The average age to reach menopause is 51, although five years either side is considered normal. This is pretty standard around the world and isn't affected by the number of pregnancies experienced or any hormonal contraception that's been taken. Even the ancient Greek philosopher Aristotle mentioned that women stopped having babies around the age of 40 to 50, so apparently the age of menopause hasn't changed for millennia. It's a natural part of the ageing process. Men also experience hormonal changes as they age, mainly involving a reduction in the production of testosterone, but the effects are generally not as sudden or dramatic as in menopause. Having said that, some people breeze through menopause without a hitch, while one in three men in their 50s will suffer serious side effects as their testosterone declines. In other words, the ageing process is an individual thing—we all experience it differently, whatever our gender.

Surgeries such as hysterectomy (removal of the uterus) and oophorectomy (removal of the ovaries), chemotherapy and radiotherapy to the pelvis can also cause menopause, regard-less of age. This is called surgical or medical menopause, and Angelina Jolie went through it after having her ovaries removed to prevent cancer.

Put simply, menopause happens when the ovaries have run out of follicles. As a quick reminder: in utero, a female foetus has about seven million follicles in the ovaries; by birth, that number has reduced to two million; by puberty, there are about 400,000. During the reproductive years, 400 to 500 mature eggs are released. By menopause, none are left.

Why the ovaries lose follicles at such high rates when so few are used is still unknown. Of course, considering millions of sperm are produced by male sex organs each day but only a few dozen make it to the fallopian tubes after ejaculation, it's not uncommon in nature to have wastage of sex cells.

Because the ovulation process has been the main source of hormone production, when there are no follicles left the ovaries reduce the production of most hormones, including oestrogen, progesterone and testosterone. Until menopause, oestrogen is the most important hormone for women, and it drops dramatically at this point, causing most of the symptoms.

But the ovaries don't power down in an orderly fashion. They become erratic: they can produce lots of oestrogen one day and none the next. As a result, periods become more irregular than usual and unpredictable, and women may suffer tender breasts, mood swings, hot flushes, night sweats, heavy bleeding and other effects.

After menopause, ovarian tissue continues to produce some oestrogen and testosterone but in smaller amounts; by then, most of the production of oestrogen and testosterone comes from fat cells and the adrenal gland.

Impacts of menopause

Most women feel some effects from menopause—a lucky 20 per cent will have none at all, and an unlucky 20 per cent will suffer severely. Effects from menopause usually last from five to ten years. The main ones are:

- hot flushes and night sweats
- mood swings
- low mood, or depression
- vaginal dryness
- lack of libido
- weight gain
- sleep problems.

I've tried to include the latest information on what menopause does to the body, but some of this remains contested while menopause remains under-researched and subject to conflicting myths, diagnoses based partly in folklore, and treatments that are far from proven to be effective.

Hot flushes and night sweats: These are simply a result of the drop in oestrogen levels. Dr Rosemary Leonard, in *Menopause: The answers*, explains: 'Changes in oestrogen levels can trigger a chain of events inside the brain, involving the chemicals serotonin and noradrenaline, that cause disruption to the working of the bit that controls your body temperature. It overreacts to just the weeniest change in temperature, and that, in turn, leads to flushes and sweats.'[29]

Mood swings and low mood: The wild fluctuation of hormones around the time of menopause is a cause of mood swings. It's believed that oestrogen has a protective effect for good mental health, and that the drop in its levels can cause low mood and depression in some women. Leonard explains: 'There are numerous oestrogen receptors throughout the brain and by acting on these this powerful hormone can influence not only mood, but also memory and concentration. There are a particularly high number of receptors in an area known as the hippocampus, which has an important role in regulating emotions. Oestrogen can also increase levels of brain neuropeptides, such as serotonin, the chemical messengers that play an important role in controlling mood, appetite and sleep.'[30]

But this doesn't fully explain the deep and often intermittent depression some people report experiencing in the perimenopause years, often referred to euphemistically as 'low mood'. As medicine becomes more acquainted with the bio-psycho-social methods of healthcare—which means looking at biological, psychological and social factors that could be causing, contributing to or affecting a condition or disease—many have tried to explain away depression at this time of life as just a coincidence. The late 40s and 50s can be busy and stressful, undoubtedly, and there doesn't seem to be adequate research to tie depression to menopause one way or the other. An Australian study found 7 per cent of women experienced depression from 45 to 54 years old, which was actually a reduction from 11 per cent in women aged eighteen to 24, and it went down to 3 per cent for women aged over 65.[31] A US study of more than 2500 women found that the majority who entered menopause didn't become depressed and those who did were more likely to have suffered depression earlier in life.[32]

This is one more area in which, sadly, not enough is known. Some women do report feeling better on some hormone replacement therapies—including those that involve testosterone—but this should be discussed with a trusted doctor.

Weight gain: Women and others with female reproductive systems change shape in their 50s, and it's not a bad thing—in fact, it's essential for good health. But as always, there's a balance. Some are shocked by their changing shape and how hard it is to lose weight, and many want a medical explanation. However, this is just nature's way of protecting you in older age. After menopause, the majority of oestrogen is produced by fat cells and the adrenal gland. You can lack the necessary oestrogen you need for good health; a little extra weight in older age, if maintained at a consistent level and not too concentrated around the waistline, protects you from a variety of conditions and extends life. What's more, a little plumpness in the cheeks helps iron out the wrinkles for people concerned about that. But, of course, there's a flip side: you can gain so much weight that additional oestrogen produced puts you at higher risk of breast and uterine cancer—not to mention a host of other chronic conditions such as diabetes and heart disease.

Sleep disturbance: The menopause years are associated with insomnia. This may be due to night sweats and hot flushes, and reduced oestrogen can also have an effect on sleep. Stress, depression and anxiety can also lead to poor sleep, and self-medicating with alcohol and caffeine will only make it worse. Lack of sleep can then lead to more stress and anxiety, and it can exacerbate aches and pains, so it's important to seek help for sleep disturbance if it's an issue.

Vaginal dryness, lack of libido and some other notes on sexuality: Let's get two points out of the way up front.

First, many women and others with female reproductive systems have wonderful sex lives well into old age, and we know that most women who had a good sex life before menopause continue to enjoy one afterwards.[33] Many women gain huge confidence and freedom in the later stages of life, and with that often comes fewer inhibitions and greater sexual enjoyment. On the other hand, some people will experience problems with a lack of interest in sex, or reduced arousal response due to vaginal and vulval dryness—but for those who see this as a problem, there are solutions, which brings me to my second point.

Lack of libido *of course* only matters if someone actually wants to have sex but finds they can't enjoy it. However, vaginal and vulval dryness can be unpleasant for anyone, whether they're having sex or not. The good news is, there are plenty of over-the-counter vaginal moisturisers on the market that can safely treat this issue. Ask your pharmacist about medically approved vaginal and vulval moisturisers and be sure not to confuse them with cosmetic cleansers and deodorants that can upset your vagina's delicate pH balance.

Vaginal dryness is mainly due to reduced oestrogen, which has an effect on moisture levels and on responses to arousal. Lack of libido is still contested ground in menopause research: it isn't recognised as an effect of menopause by the US Food and Drug Administration, and prominent endocrinologists such as the late Dr Estelle Ramey have argued menopause doesn't decrease libido at all, and that testosterone isn't reduced during and after menopause as it's produced in sufficient quantities by the adrenal gland. Studies in the UK, Denmark and Australia have all suggested that there's no correlation between menopause and lack of interest in sex.[34]

However, many medical practitioners report that some women suffer from reduced libido in the menopausal years and believe it's caused by reduced oestrogen and testosterone produced in the ovaries. Testosterone may be reduced in some post-menopausal women, and hormone therapies can affect its levels. Some studies have shown that testosterone treatment may improve sex drive in women, and an increasing number of medical practitioners believe that the hormone may help with mood and even pain reduction. However, testosterone treatment in women remains controversial.

Libido is obviously affected by enjoyment. After menopause, the vagina shrinks and loses some elasticity (this is called atrophy), and along with vaginal dryness, this could cause pain during sex, which in turn could reduce libido. Jane Ussher points to studies of lesbians that show increased sexual enjoyment compared to heterosexual women at this stage of life because they were able to discuss their body changes more openly and negotiate different ways of pleasuring each other, 'largely because they shared a broader definition of "sex" which wasn't tied to penetration'.[35]

Non-hormonal vaginal moisturisers, vaginal oestrogen therapy and/or using plenty of lubrication can improve enjoyment of sex. A pelvic physiotherapist can help if you experience pain during sex, and they can work wonders if you have incontinence issues or other generalised pelvic pain. Regular use also helps keep the vagina elastic.

It's important to remember that men are also experiencing reduced testosterone levels at this stage of their life and can start to experience sexual problems too, including reduced libido, and issues getting and maintaining an erection. And, just as women put on weight around this time, so do men. A reduced libido could also be influenced by a lack of attraction—so much has been said about women losing their looks and attractiveness after the age of 50, but attraction works two ways. And by the way, among heterosexual couples, seven out of ten divorces are instigated by women.[36] Just sayin'.

Sex drive is influenced by many factors, not just hormones, so any discussion of sexuality must look at the big picture of someone's life.

Hormone replacement therapy

Hormone therapy for menopause is nothing new. Decades before Robert Wilson published *Feminine Forever* in 1966, the US Food and Drug Administration (FDA) approved oestrogen therapy for treating the effects of menopause. And Chinese medicine has been prescribing hormone treatments for centuries: apparently wealthy women used to eat the dried urine of younger women to ease their symptoms.[37] What Wilson did, however, was classify menopause as a deficiency disease for which there was a cure, HRT, that suddenly seemed not only helpful but necessary—never mind that decreasing hormone production is a natural part of growing older for everyone.

In 1970 the late feminist and endocrinologist Dr Estelle Ramey became famous for rebutting a congressman's claim that women were unfit for important jobs because of 'raging hormonal influences'. A woman couldn't possibly be president of the USA, the congressman—a former surgeon—said: 'Suppose we had a president in the White House, a menopausal woman president who had to make the decision of the Bay of Pigs?' Ramey immediately wrote to the *Washington Star*, reminding readers that their president had, in fact, had a hormonal imbalance as he made decisions during the Cuban missile crisis: John F. Kennedy suffered from Addison's disease, in which the adrenal glands don't produce enough hormones.[38] So much is written about the effect of oestrogen on a woman's mood and her ability to think clearly; so little on the effect of testosterone on a man's mood, even though we know it can influence his ability to think clearly. Perhaps this is partly why crying is widely considered irrational and feminine, but anger is apparently rational and masculine.

The Islamic Republic of Iran has declared that women can't be judges because they're too emotional and irrational. One wonders what the Iranian ayatollahs were thinking as they watched the emotional testimony of Supreme Court

Justice Brett Kavanaugh during his selection hearings before the US Congress in September 2018.

Wilson's book quadrupled the sales of hormone replacement therapy. For decades, women were told that long-term use wasn't only safe but also protected them from a variety of diseases, including osteoporosis, heart disease and some cancers. Throughout the 1960s and 70s studies found high doses of oestrogen were causing increased risk of cardiovascular disease, stroke and endometrial cancer, so pharmaceutical companies developed lower doses and added a synthetic progesterone, progestin, to protect against endometrial cancer. They also developed better forms of hormone delivery, such as patches. By the 1980s, researchers—many sponsored by pharmaceutical companies—were claiming that oestrogen replacement in post-menopausal women could protect against Alzheimer's disease, age-related eye disease, colon cancer, tooth loss, diabetes and Parkinson's disease.[39] It was being prescribed, long-term, for any and all women, regardless of their symptoms, in order to protect them against chronic disease.

Two influential studies blew all this out of the water. A 2002 study by the US Women's Health Institute[40] and the 2003 British Million Women Study[41] found that combined oestrogen and progestin hormone therapy increased the risk of breast cancer, and the WHI study also showed it increased the risk of heart attacks and stroke. Later results from the WHI study on oestrogen-only therapy produced similar signs that risks outweighed benefits. But the breast cancer risk found in the 2002 WHI study was exaggerated by media reports, which failed to understand the meaning of relative risk and caused a great scare among women worldwide using HRT. Critics later pointed to issues with the control group in the WHI study, which had an average age of 63—much older than the typical age women are prescribed HRT.

Even taking into consideration the criticisms, together the studies showed the purported benefits of both oestrogen-only and combined hormone replacement therapy were overrated and that risks outweighed benefits in many cases. The studies helped improve scientific understanding of HRT, and medical advice changed as a result: long-term use is no longer recommended, and the benefits are considered to outweigh the risks only in women with impacts that negatively affect quality of life when started close to the date of menopause or in perimenopause, and before the age of 60. In 2013, an international group of women's health organisations worked together to review all the data on HRT; their Global Consensus Statement on Menopausal Hormone Therapy claims the benefits of taking HRT outweigh any negatives for women under 60.[42]

However, vast numbers of women continue to be both over-treated for the effects of menopause—usually wealthy women—and under-treated—usually poor and minority women.

The US FDA warns that menopausal hormone therapy isn't for everyone, and that in some women it may cause serious side effects including blood clots, heart attacks, strokes, breast cancer and gall bladder disease. While the FDA acknowledges that the therapy may help relieve hot flashes/flushes, night sweats, vaginal dryness and pain during sex, and may help protect bones, its official advice is that: 'Menopause Hormone Therapy should always be used at the lowest dose that helps and for the shortest time that you need it.'[43]

This isn't to say the controversy over HRT is settled. Some critics are still nitpicking at the Women's Health Institute and Million Women studies, and opponents of HRT claim the risks shown in these comprehensive studies are being ignored by those with an investment in selling hormone treatments.

The HRT scare that resulted from reporting on the WHI study provided a boon to a new part of the menopause industry: bioidentical hormone therapy. Proponents of this therapy claim it's natural because the hormones are derived from plants and said to be identical on a molecular level to the chemicals produced in the body. But these hormones are manufactured synthetically, like most others used in therapy, so claiming they're natural is misleading. Body-identical hormones used in HRT also have the same chemical structure as those produced in the body. As the Australian Menopause Society states: 'It is important to realise that no hormone used in any preparation of pharmaceutical grade menopausal hormone therapy (MHT) or compounded "bioidentical therapy" is "natural". They are all synthesised in the laboratory from some precursor by enzymatic manipulation.'[44]

A selling point of bioidentical hormone therapy is that treatments are individualised by testing each patient's hormone levels to develop a tailored prescription. But since hormone levels fluctuate constantly, the use of a single test is limited. The bioidentical hormone treatments compounded, or made up, by pharmacists can't be tested for safety or efficacy by regulatory agencies; this means the therapy isn't recommended as a treatment by the International Menopause Society, the North American Menopause Society, the Australasian Menopause Society or the British Menopause Society. According

to the 2016 Revised Global Consensus Statement on Menopausal Hormone Therapy: 'The use of custom-compounded
hormone therapy is not recommended because of lack of
regulation, rigorous safety and efficacy testing, batch stan-
dardisation, and purity measures.'[45]

Anyone who decides to proceed with bioidentical hormone
therapy should only do so under the care of a trusted provider
who has some qualifications in treating the effects of menopause. And the patient must accept that, as with all hormone
therapies, there are risks associated with the use of bioidentical
hormones.

Attitudes to menopause

Much is made of the fact that human beings are one of only
five mammals to go through menopause: the other four are all
whale species. New research seems to support the 'grandmother
theory' of evolution in whales, observing that grandmother
whales play an active role in the survival of their young.[46]

Pregnancy is a much more onerous process for humans
than for most other mammals, and so is raising a child. Few
mammals are as exposed to health risks during pregnancy and
childbirth as humans, and few mammalian offspring are as
helpless for as long as human children.[47] In *The Second Sex*,
Simone de Beauvoir wrote that women were 'the most deeply
alienated of all the female mammals; and she is the one that
refuses this alienation the most violently; in no other is the
subordination of the organism to the reproductive function
more imperious nor accepted with greater difficulty'.[48]

Shouldn't we then see the end of our reproductive capacity
as a great evolutionary blessing, rather than a curse?

Grace Johnston, who wrote *Menopause Essentials*, talks about her experience of menopause as a veil being lifted, allowing her to see everything in her life more clearly and giving her back energy and life focus. She adds that the post-menopause years are 'the best, happiest, and most productive time of my life'.[49]

In contrast, Rose George—a journalist who's written extensively on menopause—said of her depression during perimenopause: 'It's astonishing that I managed to shower, because I know already that this is a bad day, one when I feel assaulted by my hormones, which I picture as small pilots in those huge *Star Wars* armoured beasts that turn me this way and that, implacable.'[50] She listed other symptoms as: 'peeling skin, sore tendons, poor sleep, awful sadness, inexplicable weeping and various other "symptoms" of menopause that you can find listed if you look beyond the hot flushes and insomnia'.

A 2009 Australian study found that women assessed to have high emotional intelligence who approached menopause positively appeared to suffer less severe menopause symptoms as well as less psychological distress than women assessed to have lower emotional intelligence. The researchers concluded that 'women who expect menopause to be a negative experience or are highly stressed or distressed may be more likely to experience a more negative menopause'.[51]

After reviewing the literature and conducting in-depth interviews with sixteen Australian women, Jane Ussher concluded in *Managing the Monstrous Feminine*: 'Whilst the menopause and midlife are marked by change, at an embodied level, as well as in women's relationships, roles, and in opportunities available, and whilst ageing does bring sadness and loss, if women can tolerate the ambivalent feelings about these changes, their experiences can be positive.'[52]

If we accept that menopause is a disease, then we accept that something is wrong with it, that it isn't normal, and we surrender our bodies once again to a medical industry that's still controlled by men. Up until now, this industry has sold unproven and ineffective—and at times dangerous— treatments for menopause symptoms, and in 2019 it remains largely ignorant of the full picture of menopause and ageing in women. However, glossing over symptoms can feed into a vacuum of knowledge about sufferers' health, encouraging them to be silent and self-blaming. As Marina Benjamin argues, 'the kind of cheerleading that insists we can become strong by embracing menopause does women few favours, since it makes those of us who suffer and struggle with it feel cowed by failure and self-recrimination. We have a right to complain, damn it.'[53]

Somewhere we all have to find a happy medium where we can limit suffering without treating ageing as something that's only a disease in women. In *The Fountain of Age*, Betty Friedan wrote: 'The finding emerges that the difference between knowing and planning, and not knowing what to expect (or denial of change because of false expectations) can be the crucial factor between moving on to new growth in the last third of life, or succumbing to stagnation, pathology and despair.'[54]

As a society, we have to talk more openly and honestly about menopause at home, work (in menopause cafes, perhaps), in popular and high culture, online and in the news media. We have to know what to expect, understand that everyone who experiences menopause will have a different ride through those years, and believe that life after menopause can be exciting and fulfilling—maybe even better. We have to listen to those who welcome this stage of life as closely as we listen to those who dread it and those who suffer unpleasant effects.

We have to unpick the so-called symptoms of menopause from the normal processes of ageing, of which menopause is a part. Everyone experiences reduced hormone production as they age; everyone experiences hot flushes and night sweats, gets wrinkles, has more aches and pains and changes to hair and skin. But because menopause is tied to the uterus—the source of so much corruption!—and the female reproductive capacity, it is pathologised, turned into a condition that has to be managed by medicine.

We must also demand more research into menopause and menstruation, along with increased funding from government bodies for research into medical and non-medical treatments for ill effects these natural cycles can cause in some people's lives, and we must make sure working class and minority women and others with female reproductive systems aren't excluded or priced out of effective treatments.

Whether it's improving information about, or treatments for, the effects of menstruation or menopause, the lesson comes down to that old chestnut: we have to change society so that everyone's contributions and unique experiences are understood, accepted and valued.

CHAPTER 3

From clitoridectomy to the talking cure: a history of hysteria

Throughout history, women who haven't conformed to society's expectations of how they should behave have been written off as hysterical. Today, it's an insult usually directed at women, often in the context of them making legitimate complaints. Women are, in all Western societies, still frequently being labelled as histrionic, hysterical, emotional, difficult and mad when they present to a medical professional with complex issues. But hysteria was once a medical diagnosis, and it's from this that the insult emerged—and not by accident.

As an insult, 'hysterical' is still disarmingly effective, even when you're a world-famous athlete. Mike McRae, a science writer and the author of *Unwell*, a book on the history of disease, sums up hysteria for me simply as: 'It's a biological way of explaining why women don't act the way that we expect them to act.'

He uses Serena Williams as an example. During the 2018 US Open Women's Singles tennis final, Williams sparked global controversy by engaging in a prolonged argument with the umpire after she was given a warning for receiving instructions from her coach, effectively a charge of cheating. Williams was later penalised a point and a game as her frustration persisted; she then lost the match and was later fined US$17,000. The controversy attracted worldwide media attention, countless opinion articles and a racist cartoon published—and defended—in an Australian newspaper. While the cartoonist and newspaper denied the cartoon was racist, and just a comment on sportsmanship, news organisations and people of colour around the world disagreed with their assessment.

Williams claimed her treatment by the umpire was sexist, and here public opinion sharply divided. Were the penalties dished out to her more severe because she wasn't acting as a woman is supposed to? Would a man have received such harsh penalties if he'd acted the same way? Race issues can't be ignored, either, since the anger of a black woman is interpreted by mainstream Western society as more aggressive and threatening than anger from a white woman, or even perhaps a white man. As professor of law at Duke Law School in the US, Trina Jones—who has studied how racial stereotyping affects the lives of African American women—told the BBC at the time: 'Black women are not supposed to push back and when they do, they're deemed to be domineering. Aggressive. Threatening. Loud.'[1]

While the issues raised over the incident are complex, McRae thinks it's a good example of how ideas about hysteria remain embedded in our society. I spoke to him just after the event, and he said, 'There's a lot of controversy around

[Serena Williams] not acting as you would expect a woman to act on the tennis court. And you see the word "hysterical" come up quite often. If you saw a man behaving that way—and quite often we've seen male tennis players throw their racket around and question things—you wouldn't hear the word "hysterical" being applied. You wouldn't look to a male tennis player and go, "They're being a little too emotional". Because we already think he is behaving in a reasonable way.'

Because male anger and aggression are considered normal, they're not seen as out of character or, in many cases, offensive or confronting when acted out, especially during a sports match. White men are presumed reasonable, so how they act isn't questioned. But women are considered emotional, ruled by their hormones and irrational—so when they act outside of accepted feminine roles, their very sanity is questioned.

Is it really hysterical or even unreasonable to question a charge of cheating, especially when it happens often in tennis and Williams insists she didn't see the coach instructing her? And was the rage of a woman—one of the greatest athletes of all time—really not understandable when you consider the microaggressions committed against her over the decades she's been a tennis champion? Her looks, weight, muscles, strength and femininity have been subjected to constant criticism and abuse; rarely her ability or athleticism, which remain unquestionable. It's worth noting that Williams was playing in a bespoke tutu after the French Open banned her black catsuit—which had also been custom-designed to protect her from blood clots that she'd experienced after childbirth—saying, 'One must respect the game and the place.'[2]

Let's look at another example. In this case, it's of a woman having an opinion. Witness this exchange between two Australians on ABC TV's *Q&A*: TV and radio host Steve Price, and writer and *Guardian* columnist Van Badham. A male audience member, whose sister had been murdered by her male partner asked the panel, which also included several members of parliament, how politicians and the media could play a better role in shifting the language around violence against women. That week, some sports commentators had created a national controversy for joking about drowning a female sports journalist on their show. Steve Price was first to respond and spent his time making excuses for the men at the centre of the controversy. They were 'a bunch of blokes laughing about something they shouldn't have laughed about', he said, and added: 'I think too much was made of what was originally a joke on a football show.' He didn't address the man's question or the horrific murder of the questioner's sister or talk about the statistics that show one woman is murdered by an intimate partner every week in Australia, or how media narratives feed into a culture that excuses violence against women. Van Badham was asked to respond next. She began, 'What you see as jokes made by a bunch of blokes—from the position of one of those blokes who's probably been in on one of those jokes—I see—as a woman who is part of a social world where violence is . . .'

There, Price interrupts her, objecting to the suggestion he'd ever been in on such a joke. Badham says she wasn't suggesting that and tries to carry on to make her point. For the next minute, Price continues to interrupt Badham, she can't get out more than a dozen words without being interrupted by him until eventually the host intervenes and asks Price to let Badham finish.

HOST: Steve, I'll give you a chance to respond in a moment but Van . . .

VB: Thank you, you are proving my point very excellently about the attitudes that create this kind of . . .

SP [interrupts]: I don't think I'm proving any point at all.

VB: . . . problem.

AUDIENCE CLAPS and CHEERS

VB: So I think we need to bring up [that] the challenges are multifaceted. One, we have to stop creating these binary . . . men are this, women are this. Masculinity is this, femininity is this. Men have high status, women have low status. You can speak down to these people but these people are not allowed to speak back up. That we can make jokes, and oh yeah it's all jokes and they apologised and that's fine but on the receiving end is the ludicrous proportion of women who do experience violence . . .

SP [interrupts]: I think you're just being hysterical.

AUDIENCE GROANS

VB: It's probably my ovaries making me do it, Steve.[3]

Why does that taunt still sting? And how did this come to be? What was hysteria when it was considered a disease, and why are we finding it so hard to expel hysteria from our culture—not just in medicine but in society's ideas about women? I think it becomes much easier to understand when we look at the history of hysteria. In understanding the origins of this enigmatic disease, we can more clearly see how it transformed from an idea about woman as a walking womb—which was itself insatiable, 'an animal within an animal'[4]—to witches, to hysteria as an organic disease, to one of mental illness or madness. The word 'hysteria' has always been shorthand for 'difficult women'.

As cultural historian George Rousseau and others have observed: in every generation, hysteria is mainly a reflection of that society's culture, in particular its ideas about gender and class, and women's roles within those structures. 'Hysteria is a unique phenomenon in the entire repertoire of Western medicine,' wrote Rousseau in *Hysteria Beyond Freud*, 'because it exposes the traditional binary components of the medical model—mind/body, pathology/normalcy, health/sickness, doctor/patient—as no other condition ever has.'[5]

A HISTORY OF HYSTERIA

Woman's difference has always marked her as inferior. The uterus—the most obvious mark of difference—was once considered the source of all disease. Then, in the seventeenth century, the source of women's illness shifted from the uterus to her weak 'nervous system', before shifting back to the reproductive system: this time to the ovaries and clitoris. After the discovery of sex hormones in the early twentieth century, it shifted again, this time to her 'raging hormones'. Through all these shifts in blame, society's distrust of women remained constant.

In the beginning

'Hysteria' comes from the Greek word for the uterus, *hystera*, but contrary to popular belief 'hysteria' as a diagnosable condition doesn't come from Hippocrates. Born in 460 BC in Classical Greece, Hippocrates is considered the Father of Medicine; he was the first to propose that disease is an organic problem within the body and not a punishment from the gods. Some of his principles live on today, but the volume of medical theory known as the Hippocratic corpus wasn't written by him, as so long believed, but by a collection of physicians over many years. His most famous contribution to modern medicine is the Hippocratic Oath, which governs the ethics of doctors—again, he didn't write it himself.

While Hippocrates didn't invent hysteria as we now understand it, the British classical scholar Helen King has shown how his work influenced its development as a condition up until the early modern era.[6] Till then, physicians practised according to ideas largely developed by the Hippocratic corpus, and by later Greek physicians such as Soranus and Galen in Roman times. All illness was seen as systemic, and cures required physicians to decipher where the balance of the patient's internal system had been lost and how to re-establish it. There was no separation between a malady of the body or mind.

In *Hysteria: The disturbing history,* Andrew Scull wrote: 'Women were different. Of that there could be no doubt. And the differences were consequential for their health. Hence the disposition of physicians in the ancient world to place women's reproductive systems at the heart of accounting for their susceptibility to all sorts of disease and debility. In women, so one Hippocratic text read, "the womb is the origin of all diseases".'[7]

Puberty, menstruation, pregnancy, childbirth and menopause were all viewed with suspicion, treated as illnesses and said to account for almost any ill a woman suffered. The Greek philosopher Plato, and many others after him, believed the uterus wandered around the body in search of moisture and in need of fertilisation. In Plato's dialogue, *Timaeus*, c. 360 BC, the womb is 'voracious, predatory, appetitive, unstable, forever reducing the female into a frail and unstable creature', according to Rousseau. In the first century AD Aretaeus of Cappadocia built on Plato's ideas, and feared the wandering womb could slip into other body parts and suffocate its owner. He referred to it as an 'animal within an animal'[8] and his treatment was to use nice-smelling fragrances via water steaming placed at the vulva to coax it back into place. He called the condition *hysterike pnix*, or 'suffocation caused by the womb'.[9]

In the following centuries, the medical texts developed by these men travelled from West to East and back again: they were interpreted, added to and translated from Greek to Arabic, and returned to the West via Latin in the fifteenth and sixteenth centuries. While medical knowledge grew, and the invention of dissection meant the notion of the 'wandering womb' could be discounted, it's amazing how the old stories lived on and came to form the roots of hysteria as we now understand it.

Treatments dreamt up in ancient times such as vaginal steaming, bandaging to keep the uterus in place, inducing sneezes, and 'bloodletting' by leeches on the cervix or labia, or by doctors extracting blood from the patient, all remained firm beliefs in the medical texts. It was thought female illness could at once be caused by lack of sex, but also too much sex, or merely desiring it. Pregnancy was frequently offered as a cure for all manner of ills.

So here's the origin of the uterus as a thing that lives apart from the woman—a being that can be blamed for almost any female malady, rooted in ancient history. By the Middle Ages, the Hippocratic texts had been largely abandoned in the West. But that didn't make things easier for women. In the late Middle Ages and early modern era, so-called difficult women who refused to conform to the feminine ideal—often with symptoms that would later be defined as hysteria—were more likely to be declared witches and burnt at the stake. It's estimated that between 40,000 and 60,000 accused witches were killed in Europe between 1400 and 1782. While some men were accused of witchcraft, the majority were women.[10]

Seventeenth century: the medicalisation of hysteria

In 1603, a woman called Elizabeth Jackson was put on trial in England for bewitching the fourteen-year-old girl, Mary Glover. An eminent physician, Edward Jorden, appeared as a witness to proclaim that Glover wasn't possessed by the devil but was suffering from a physical condition called *hysteria passio* or 'suffocation of the mother', terms that would become inter-changeable with 'hysteria' through the seventeenth century. Jorden didn't believe it was a result of a wandering womb but nevertheless believed in the womb's close connections with the brain, heart and liver, and its effects on the veins, arteries and nerves. The jury didn't buy Jorden's theory and Jackson was convicted of witchcraft, but Jorden persisted. At the request of the Bishop of London, he wrote a pamphlet about this condition, *hysteria passio*, urging people to recognise that symptoms usually viewed as possession were in fact a physical disease originating in the uterus. Rooted in Hippocratic and Galenic tradition, Jorden's theory didn't hold much sway over his fellow physicians at the start of the century, but the pamphlet has been given some credit for helping to end the legal persecution of witches[11] and as a herald of the hysteria to come.

Around the same time Jorden was developing his theories, a Dutch physician called Johannes Wier concluded that the largely female malady of love sickness, which had been prevalent through the Middle Ages, was caused by the uterus. It was believed that women had seed, similar to sperm, which if not expelled by orgasm could become poisonous and lead to symptoms commonly associated with hysteria; both too much purging of the seed (too much sex) and too much retention (not enough sex) were considered harmful. Heterosexual sex within marriage was thought to be the only cure. Wier, a sympathetic physician, cared deeply about his patients' suffering.

Jorden and Wier believed they were doing a great service to the women accused of witchcraft by arguing that the signs and symptoms were the result of a disease rather than the devil. It took many decades for other doctors to agree with the two physicians. By the mid-1600s, the very symptoms that possessed Mary Glover: 'loss of speech and sight, an inability to swallow; paralyses of hands, arms and legs; mysterious swellings of the abdomen or throat; a sense of suffocation; odd breathing patterns; loss of sensation and of reflex action'[12] would be widely known as the symptoms of hysteria.

In the 1680s, English physicians Thomas Willis and Thomas Sydenham completed the medicalisation of hysteria and influenced how it would be perceived for centuries to come. Sydenham, known as the English Hippocrates for his meticulous observation of patients, treated thousands of hysterics, rich and poor, in his busy London clinic. He is, according to Rousseau, the unacknowledged 'hero of hysteria'[13] for his four prescient observations of the disease: he was the first to declare that both women and men could be hysterical (though most patients were still women), to observe it was a 'disease of civilisation', to declare it wasn't a disease of the uterus, and to name it the most common of all diseases among women.[14] In naming hysteria a disease of civilisation, what Sydenham meant was that the richer a person was, the more demanding life was, and so the more likely they were to become hysterical. He believed the social conditions that enslaved women caused inner turmoil that resulted in physical illness—an observation ahead of its time.

While Sydenham developed his ideas through observations of his many patients, Thomas Willis developed his through a study of medical theory. He also believed both men and women could be hysterical but, unlike Sydenham, he thought the disease emanated mainly from the uterus as it radiated through the nervous system. By the end of the seventeenth century, hysteria was considered primarily a disease of the nervous system, though Willis didn't develop ideas on how the male reproductive system influenced hysteria in men.

Although both Willis and Sydenham in theory believed hysteria could affect men, it was still primarily a female condition and diagnosed only in effeminate men, those who were thought to have weak nervous systems in common with women. Usually, men were being diagnosed with a separate but similar condition known as melancholy.

Many doctors at the time were unsympathetic to

hysterical patients, dismissing their symptoms as fake and so much attention-seeking, but Sydenham and Willis believed in the physical pain of their patients and worked hard to alleviate their suffering. In doing so, they medicalised hysteria—and while its symptoms and causes changed over the follow-ing centuries, the essential idea of the condition did not. As Rousseau wrote, 'If we ask what the three hundred years between 1500 and 1800 can teach us about hysteria, the answer can be found by looking at two factors: gender-based pain and social conditions, neither of which falls within accepted cate-gories of modern medicine.'[15]

Eighteenth century: hysteria is a disease of the nervous system
English life changed dramatically from the late 1600s to 1800. London's population grew from 300,000 in 1660, to 675,000 in 1700, to over a million in 1800. Urbanisation was happen-ing for the first time, violent crime increased and the suffering caused by poverty was being realised. It was a time of profound stress for women. The industrial revolution had appeared to offer them greater freedom but society failed to accept women who wanted roles outside the home. As society changed in new and interesting ways, social isolation and punishment grew for upper class women who took time away from their children to develop their own interests.

Throughout the next two centuries, it wasn't just doctors labelling otherwise well women as hysterical: women presented themselves to doctors with the symptoms of hysteria, begging for a diagnosis. They wanted their condition to be recognised as a genuine disease—and they wanted a treatment that would make them feel better.

By the eighteenth century, medical theory had firmly rooted hysteria in the nervous system. Apparently the greater susceptibility of women was owing to their weaker nerves, which was put down to their excess blood—the animalistic womb had been discarded but a woman's bodily functions as a source of suspicion and infection had not.

If hysteria had grown common by the end of the seventeenth century, it became epidemic in the eighteenth. An explosion in scientific knowledge across Europe encouraged doctors to promote medicine as a science. No influential doctor still believed the uterus was the cause of disease, and the idea that physical symptoms might be induced in the brain was inconceivable. Physicians and philosophers were bringing a mathematical focus to understanding the human body, and deciphering how the nervous system worked was a big part of that. By the last third of the century, it was understood that nerves carried signals around the body to and from the brain. Diseases of the nervous system, with all its complications, gave physicians' diagnoses creditability at a time when doctors were trying to distinguish themselves from charlatans and quacks.[16]

Hysteria's status as a disease of the nervous system had given it legitimacy, making it a somewhat desirable diagnosis, as opposed to ill-defined conditions such as the vapours, melancholy and hypochondria. John Radcliffe was dismissed as Queen Anne's doctor in the 1690s when he diagnosed her with the vapours, which was by then thought to be imaginary—patients wanted diagnoses of bodily illnesses that could be treated with pharmacological prescriptions. Then, as now, patients wanted their pain taken seriously, to be believed, and to have something to blame for their misery.

That's when George Cheyne came along, dismissing as nonsense ideas that animal spirits governed the nervous system and that humours balanced humans' inner bodies. Like Sydenham, Cheyne put forward hysteria as a disease of civilisation. In his 1733 book *The English Malady*, he argues that far from being a condition to be ashamed of, hysteria was evidence of the success of English industrialisation. Cheyne and other Enlightenment doctors had genuine sympathy for their patients, not least because they were gleaned from the rich and famous; hysteria was a thorn in the side of 'elites moving in flashy, fast-lane society', the 'victims of an interestingly delicate nervous system buckling under the pressures of civilization'.[17] Treatments included bleeding and blistering, as well as diet, exercise, rest and diversion: all preserves of the rich.

Madness was still a personal failing, but hysteria was a sign of accomplishment. Even so, it remained a largely female condition, and men began to resist the diagnosis by the end of the century. Some Western women had a glimpse of freedom. Movements such as the Blue Stockings Society in England— founded in the 1750s, it advocated for education and counted women authors, scandalous at the time, among its numbers— flourished for a while, but little progress was made in women's social conditions. Universities were still closed to women, their education limited. In Europe at least, women were still walking wombs, and the only way to prevent a woman's fragile nerves from developing into hysteria was to conform to the 'prevailing social and biological notions of womanhood'.[18] The fact that male doctors claimed hysteria could be a male and female disease but reserved diagnosis for women made the weaker female seem natural—her nervousness, sexual desire and confinement to the home were unchangeable facts and God-given decrees.

Under these conditions we meet the German doctor, Franz Anton Mesmer. He was as staunch a believer in new scientific principles as his English counterparts and subscribed to the prevailing theories of the nervous system. But while others argued over the mechanisms by which nerves carried signals to and from the brain, he claimed to have identified a different nerve force. Called animal magnetism, it was completely natural and could cure all manner of ills, chiefly hysteria, and some people—namely, him—had the power to transform it from one being to another. He could do it through a simple gaze, or by laying his hands on a body, or by running his hands over the body without even touching it, or by filling a tub with iron filings and allowing patients to touch rods protruding from the tub, which allowed mass healings to take place.[19] Animal magnetism unblocked disease-causing obstructions in the body, he preached, and allowed energy to flow freely.

Mesmer moved to Paris in 1778 and while opinion was split on whether he was a genius or a fake, his reputation as a charismatic healer spread in Parisian high society and he counted French aristocracy among his patients. Mesmer began appearing at mass healings wearing a lavender silk robe and occasionally playing a glass harp. His colleagues, however, were deaf to his charms and scornful of his practice, saying his gatherings were sexual and debauched. He was never accepted into the Royal Academy of Sciences or the Royal Society of Medicine but his influential patients defended him staunchly, and eventually the King commissioned the Royal Academy to assess his practices. Benjamin Franklin, then the American ambassador to France, was among the academy members to conclude that animal magnetism was nothing more than a figment of Mesmer's and his patients' imaginations and animal magnetism was largely forgotten.

But hysteria became further entrenched in French misogynistic culture during the Revolution, and by the end of the century, patriarchal society had strengthened.

Nineteenth century: a battle between gynaecology and neurology

This century saw theories of hysteria ping pong from a disease of the nervous system, to one of corrupted female sex organs, back to the nervous system and finally into a psychological malady, creating the conditions for Sigmund Freud to develop his now famous psychological theories and techniques.

It's also the century during which gynaecology and neurology became medical specialities, in no small part because of their claims to own the treatment for hysteria. As if to broadcast that hysteria was just another method of social control, it became linked with feminist movements as the nineteenth century ended.

This too was the century in which lunatic asylums became widespread. While madness or lunacy wasn't yet gendered as a diagnosis, often the only difference between women diagnosed as mad and those diagnosed as hysterics was their wealth. A new speciality was created—what we now call psychiatry. These doctors were often looked down upon by other physicians but asylums spread throughout Europe and America.

For all these reasons—and more—how hysteria was treated in the late nineteenth and early twentieth century is of real interest for us now. During this time, according to Barbara Ehrenreich and Deirdre English, medicine became an elite profession and took over from religious institutions as the primary enforcers of the social roles of women. This period, they write in *Complaints and Disorders*, 'witnessed a pronounced shift from a religious to a biomedical rationale for sexism, as well as the formation of the medical profession as we know it—a male elite with a legal monopoly over medical practice'.[20]

In the early 1800s, hysterics were still big business for general practitioners. Treatments for hysteria were dominated by bleeding (either by lancet, cupping or leeches), pills, nerve tonics, iron, arsenic, opiates and vomiting, as well as a change of scenery or bathing in sulphurous waters, such as at the resort town of Bath or in the many spas popping up all over Germany.[21] And if all that failed, they could now be transferred to an asylum.

'In general,' the feminist writer and literary critic Elaine Showalter wrote, 'Victorian doctors saw hysteria as a disorder of female adolescence, caused both by the establishment of the menses and by the development of sexual feelings that could have no outlet or catharsis.'[22] Unlike men, women had no work, physical exercise or intellectual pursuits—no way to release the abundance of emotion and energy produced during puberty—and this fostered hysteria in them, the theory went. The condition reflected gender roles by situating a male doctor in charge of an overly emotional woman, but hysteria has also been seen as a protest by women at their limited roles in nineteenth-century life. 'Reared to be weak, dependent, flirtatious, and unassertive, many American girls grew up to be child-women, unable to cope with the practical and emotional demands of adult life. They defended themselves against the hardships and obligations of adulthood "by regressing towards the childish hyper-femininity of the hysteric".'[23] In 1911 the feminist writer Charlotte Perkins Gilman, a diagnosed hysteric, wrote that American men 'have bred a race of women who are physically weak enough to be handed about like invalids; or mentally weak enough to pretend they are— and to like it'.[24]

Doctors eventually became fed up with the interminable queues of hysterical women who filled their waiting rooms and never seemed to get better. A certain kind of malice emerged in the way physicians wrote about their hysterical patients and in the harshness of the remedies offered. It didn't help that women complained of not being cured, and went from doctor to doctor in search of better treatments. One such man, W. Tyler Smith, treated his nervous and menopausal patients 'by a course of injections of ice water into the rectum, introduction of ice into the vagina, and leeching of the labia and cervix'.[25]

Another young doctor, Robert Brudenell Carter—who would later abandon treating hysterics—described his hostility to hysterical women in an 1853 book, *On the Pathology and Treatment of Hysteria*. He believed that while a physical disease may have induced an initial fit, most hysterics were faking their severe symptoms, and only the harshest treatment could force them out of it. The benefits of being sick were so great—in terms of the power it gave them at home—Carter and other doctors believed women were willing to suffer immensely to keep up the charade. Carter thought the condition also involved sexual repression and that these women were severely morally depraved, their persistence with illness the result of 'selfishness and deceptivity'.[26] He wrote: 'I have . . . seen young unmarried women, of the middle classes of society, reduced, by the constant use of the speculum, to the mental and moral condition of prostitutes; seeking to give themselves the same indulgence by the practice of solitary vice; and asking every medical practitioner, under whose care they fell, to institute an examination of the sexual organs.'[27] His prescribed treatment involved a severe form of psychotherapy, which asked the patient to picture herself, with the help of a 'speaker' who would raise 'any and every part of her past conduct, which can conduce to her humiliation and shame'[28] to encourage recovery.

Carter was only 25 years old when he wrote his book. The fact that few women would sign up for his harsh and insensitive treatment may have been one of the reasons he lost interest in treating hysterics.

Gynaecology's brutal surgical experiments

While the nervous system continued to play a central role in theories of hysteria, the female reproductive system again took centre stage in the long battle to understand this mysterious condition during the nineteenth century.

The Victorian age was the pinnacle of hysteria diagnoses, and for doctors nothing was clearer than that a woman was, as Carroll Smith-Rosenberg and Charles Rosenberg put it, 'the product and prisoner of her reproductive system'.[29] Women's limited role in society was positioned as natural, therefore unchangeable. It wasn't because men wanted women at home subservient to them—it was this way because nature intended it, because women's reproductive systems demanded it.

George Man Burrows, an English 'mad doctor', was pivotal in the development of the reflex theory. He claimed science showed that women's brains and reproductive systems were so closely linked, any disruption in one could wreak havoc on the other.[30] Puberty, menstruation, pregnancy, childbirth, lactation and menopause all put such strain on a woman and created such shocks in her system that they accounted for no end of mental disturbances, weak emotions, low intelligence, loss of self-control and greater susceptibility to nervous illnesses such as hysteria. Sex outside of marriage, desiring too much sex within marriage, masturbation or just sexual thoughts could all provoke a shock big enough to induce illness, even insanity. As working-class women entered the ranks of the hysterics, their greater propensity to satisfy their most animal-istic desires—proven by their higher birth rates—was given as justification for the reflex theory.

Around the middle of the century, gynaecology began to develop as a specialist medical practice. Gynaecologists/obstetricians would be present at childbirth, and they also made themselves responsible for treating hysteria. Surgical techniques advanced with the discovery of anaesthesia in the 1840s and the promotion of antiseptics in the last third of the century—and these advances were put to use in childbirth. Women had traditionally worked as midwives and healers, so the reflex theory worked well for the men in this emerging profession by finding a biological reason for kicking women out of it. Ehrenreich and English wrote: 'For the doctors, the myth of female frailty thus served two purposes. It helped them to disqualify women as healers, and, of course, it made women highly qualified as patients.'[31]

Englishman Isaac Baker Brown was a leading gynaecologist of the time. In the 1850s, he was the first to use chloroform as an anaesthetic in childbirth. He developed new techniques for repairing vaginal and anal fistulae, and prolapsed uteruses—all complications of childbirth.

Baker Brown soon became a celebrity and was praised in *The Lancet*. He decided conclusively that hysteria was caused by masturbation, which led to a loss of nerve power, in turn leading to hysteria.[32] His cure was the surgical removal of the clitoris. He wasn't the first physician in Western civilisation to propose this: Soranus of Ephesus had also recommended it in the second century in cases of 'oversized clitorises, lest they cause women to take on a more dominant role in sex or worse still, reject men altogether'.[33] Between 1858 and 1866 Baker Brown performed many clitoridectomies, which he declared an unmitigated success in an 1866 book.[34]

Within a year of the book's release, however, Baker Brown was cast out from the profession, and his operations ceased. This ostracism wasn't due to the sadistic nature of his treatment but rather because his relentless pursuit of publicity made the practice of medicine look almost like a working-class trade at a time when doctors were trying to establish themselves as elite professionals.

In proposing to expel Baker Brown from the Obstetrical Society, its vice-president Sir Francis Seymour Haden wrote: 'we have constituted ourselves, as it were, the guardians of [women's] interests, and in many cases . . . the custodians of their honour. We are, in fact, the stronger, and they the weaker. They are obliged to believe all that we tell them. They are not in a position to dispute anything we say to them, and we therefore may be said to have them at our mercy.'[35]

Before settling on the clitoridectomy as a cure for hysteria, Baker Brown had experimented with surgery to remove the ovaries, resulting in the deaths of his first three patients. But towards the end of the 1800s surgical death rates had declined, paving the way for another gynaecologist to propose yet another cure for female ills. The American surgeon Robert Battey announced in 1873 that the removal of the ovaries could induce early menopause and cure hysteria along with other menstrual and nervous disorders. He wasn't the first surgeon to remove the ovaries but he was the first to systematically remove healthy ovaries for a variety of non-gynaecological symptoms.[36]

By 1886, surgical methods were so improved that Battey reported only two deaths in his 70 surgeries, which came to be known as Battey's operations, now called oophorectomy.

It isn't known exactly how many of these surgeries were performed but the records show at least several thousand and possibly tens of thousands of women had their healthy ovaries removed in the last two decades of the nineteenth century. It seems the surgery was more popular in the United States than Europe.

Many but not all doctors were on board with the surgery, although again the critics' disagreement wasn't based on the cruelty of the treatment: this time it was the surgery's effect on women's social roles. What use was a woman who couldn't reproduce, these enlightened physicians argued? And there was a word for women who'd have sex without the chance of procreation. Nobody would marry her.

Following the American Civil War in the 1860s, a new group of doctors had risen to prominence in the United States. They called themselves neurologists and laid claim to the latest science regarding the nervous system, and they were the most harshly critical of the oophorectomy. In 1893, A.M. Hamilton wrote in the *New Medical Journal* that it was 'heroic surgery, of . . . the most flagrant and pernicious form';[37] in 1896, neurologist R.T. Edes wrote in the *Journal of the American Medical Association* that the surgery's 'evil and uselessness can not be too strongly condemned'.[38] In 1896, Howard Kelly from Johns Hopkins School of Medicine, the leading gynaecologist of his age, wrote in the *Journal of the American Medical Association* that the surgery was 'the destroyer of everything that makes a woman's life worth living'.[39] By the mid-1890s, elite gynaecologists were mostly opposed to the surgery, and it declined in popularity.

Once again, doctors had placed themselves as the moral and medical guardians of women and their place in society.

Neurology

While there had been nerve doctors in Europe and America in the previous century, US neurology grew as a force as its proponents responded to a new class of patient: men wounded in the American Civil War. Some of them had traumatic injuries of the brain, spinal cord and nervous system, and many had other nervous complaints resembling hysteria.

The neurologists' focus on the brain and nervous system meant they treated all forms of mental disease. Clear distinctions between neurological and psychiatric diseases had not yet been drawn, and the neurologists positioned themselves as scientifically superior to the asylum doctors. Soon, it wasn't just male war veterans filling the waiting rooms of these new doctors, but middle- and upper-class men too.

Throughout history, whenever growing numbers of men with hysteria-like symptoms showed up to doctors' rooms, a new condition would be invented to account for it. Neurasthenia was named in the 1870s by the American neurologist George Beard, who declared it a disease of nervous exhaustion—unlike hysteria, though, neurasthenia had the mark of respect. And just as Cheyne had declared hysteria a sign of English accomplishment, so Beard described neurasthenia as a disease of American civilisation, superiority and success.

According to neurologists, only the most accomplished people suffered from neurasthenia: bankers, lawyers, titans of industry—people who worked more with their brains than their hands. Or as Beard wrote: 'the civilised, refined and educated', not 'the barbarous and low-born and untrained'.[40] Beard had suffered a nervous collapse, so he counted himself among its sufferers; one in ten neurasthenics were doctors, he claimed.

In reality, the symptoms of neurasthenia and hysteria were the same. At first there wasn't a clear gender divide in hysteria and neurasthenia—women were diagnosed as neurasthenics and men as hysterics. But, as the century wore on, diagnoses of neurasthenia favoured men and hysteria women.

In the second half of the nineteenth century, doctors developed a new theory centred on the conservation of energy that conveniently justified the limited social roles of women. Humans are born with a finite store of energy, the theory went, and those who use too much of it simply break down. Neurasthenia and hysteria reflected the overuse or abuse of the brain, stomach or reproductive system. Darwin's 1871 publication of *The Descent of Man, and Selection in Relation to Sex* supposedly provided scientific proof that women were inferior to men and naturally inclined to domestic duties.

Edward Clark in the United States and Henry Maudsley in England argued that mental and physical energy were finite and competing: 'What Nature spends in one direction, she must economise in another direction,' Maudsley wrote.[41] And because the female reproductive system expended so much energy, women should focus solely on their roles as mothers-to-be. These ideas were used to justify keeping girls out of school, away from any athletic pursuits and in the home, reproducing. Elaine Showalter explains: 'The higher education of women in universities was obviously then a threat not only to their health but to their reproductive capacities . . . and so the young woman who gave herself over to learning would find her sexual and reproductive organs atrophying, her "pelvic power" diminished or destroyed, and her fate one of sexlessness and disease.'[42]

A leading American neurologist of the day, Silas Weir Mitchell, developed the notorious rest cure in the late 1800s as a treatment for hysteria and neurasthenia. A strong critic of American universities such as Vassar that had begun educating women, Mitchell was known for despising his female hysterical patients. He said, 'a hysterical girl is a vampire who sucks the blood of the healthy people around her'.[43] He nevertheless believed it was a real condition of the nervous system and that it could be cured through enforced rest and feeding. 'The rest cure evolved from Mitchell's work with "malingering" soldiers in the Civil War, whom he had assigned to the most disagreeable jobs, so that after a few weeks in the latrines they were eager to return,' wrote Showalter.[44]

The rest cure became hugely popular in the United States and Europe, and Mitchell counted some famous women as his patients, including Jane Addams, Edith Wharton and Charlotte Perkins Gilman, who made its cruelty famous in her short-story 'The Yellow Wallpaper'. The cure involved the patient being confined to bed for six weeks and cared for by a nurse not known or related to them, while they were fed continuously with a high-fat diet and received massages and electric treatments to encourage digestion and stimulate the bowels; urine and faeces were passed lying down. For one hour a day, the patient—usually female because they were more likely to accept, or be coerced into accepting, the treatment—could be lifted onto a lounge while the bed was changed. No reading, writing or mental stimulation was allowed. Virginia Woolf received a modified version of the rest cure in 1904 and was said to despise it.

Only the rich could afford the rest cure. What working-class woman could take to bed for six weeks while paying a nurse to feed her a rich diet and massage her constantly? But working-class men and women nonetheless were increasingly presenting with nervous disorders.

Jean-Martin Charcot

The French physician Jean-Martin Charcot deserves his own heading partly because of his highly questionable treatment of hysteria and his medical accomplishments outside of it, as well as the inspiration he provided to Sigmund Freud. Photos of his elaborate public exhibitions of his female hysterical patients, likened to a circus, became the lasting images of nineteenth-century hysteria.

Working in the last few decades of the 1800s, Charcot was a leading neurologist of the era, and he grew rich treating European royalty and newly minted merchants. His many accomplishments in internal medicine and neurology included identifying diseases such as multiple sclerosis, aphasia, amyotrophic lateral sclerosis (ALS, known as motor neurone disease in Australia and the UK; in France it's Charcot's disease), locomotor ataxia (a complication of tertiary syphilis), Tourette's syndrome, Charcot-Marie-Tooth disorder and chorea.[45] He was put in charge of the Salpêtrière, originally a gunpowder factory that was converted to a hospice for Paris's outcast, abandoned and unwell women in 1656 by Louis XIV. It became a teaching hospital attached to the Sorbonne and, with a capacity of 10,000 patients, was one of the world's largest hospitals when Charcot was there. The position provided Charcot with captive patients, the ability to study them over a long period and perform autopsies on them.

Charcot declared hysteria a disorder of the nervous system, not the female reproductive system. This stole ground from the French gynaecologists performing oophorectomies. And while his version of hysteria wasn't a disease of the reproductive system, it retained its sexual element. As George Rousseau noted in *Hysteria Beyond Freud*: 'Women who complained of chronic pain that could not be located in the nervous system ran the risk of finding themselves classified as hypochondriacs suffering from imaginary illnesses. What had presented itself to the Greeks as a fiery animal, an overheated, labile, voracious, and raging uterus, was now, in Charcot's world, diagnosed as a sexually diseased and morally debauched female imagination.'[46]

He believed *le gran de hystérie* followed a pattern in three stages: 'the epileptoid phase in which the patient lost conscious-ness and foamed at the mouth; the phase of "clownism" (Charcot was a great fan of the circus), involving eccentric physical contortions; and the phase of "attitudes passionnelles", or sexual poses. The attack ended with a back-bend called the *arc-en-cercle*.'[47] Charcot believed he could cure it with hypnosis, which he demonstrated in front of audiences comprised of the Parisian elite. The demonstrations became renowned for the writhing and moaning of the patients, the sexual under-tone of which both attracted and repelled the crowds.

A Swedish doctor, Axel Munthe, who was practising in Paris and attended one of Charcot's performances, later described it: 'The huge amphitheatre was filled to the last place with a multicoloured audience drawn from tout Paris, authors, journalists, leading actors and actresses, fashionable demimondaines.' Charcot would appear on stage with hypno-tised women: 'some of them smelt with delight a bottle of ammonia when told it was rose water, others would eat a piece of charcoal when presented to them as chocolate. Another would crawl on all fours on the floor, barking furiously when told she was a dog, flap her arms as if trying to fly when turned into a pigeon, lift her skirts with a shriek of terror when a glove was thrown at her feet with a suggestion of being a snake. Another would walk with a top hat in her arms rocking it to and fro and kissing it tenderly when told it was a baby.'[48]

Despite his notoriety and power to silence dissent, Charcot had his critics—and some were very high-profile, including the writers Tolstoy and de Maupassant. The Belgian feminist writer and activist Madame Céline Renooz wrote in *Revue scientifique des femmes* that his treatment was a 'sort of vivisection of women under the pretext of studying a disease for which he knows neither the cause nor the treatment'.[49]

It would be too easy to write off Charcot as just another misogynist whose interest lay in upholding the status quo along both gender and class lines. In fact, he believed that women should be educated to the highest levels, he trained some female doctors, and he argued that the working classes had the same constitutions as the middle and upper classes. He did, however, see hysteria in strictly gendered terms; as the American historian Mark Micale wrote, 'Women in his writings fell ill due to their vulnerable emotional natures and inability to control their feelings, while men got sick from working, drinking, and fornicating too much. Hysterical women suffered from an excess of "feminine" behaviors, hysterical men from an excess of "masculine" behaviors.'[50]

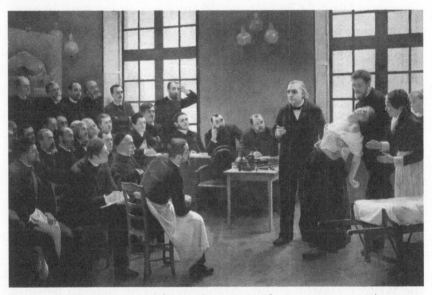

Photos taken at Charcot's elaborate hypnotic performances came to be seen as the defining images of hysteria. This 1887 painting by André Brouillet shows one of Charcot's lectures.

But Charcot's thin skin meant he was surrounded by yes-men, so scared of upsetting him that they staged his exhibitions without question. There never was a typical three-stage fit among hysterics, and when he died in 1892 the whole edifice came crumbling down as former protégés became critics and admitted their deception—of Charcot as well as the crowds. By 1900, hysteria had largely disappeared as a diagnosis in Paris.

Sigmund Freud

None of this persuaded a young Sigmund Freud to disown Charcot's theories. After studying under him for four months from 1885 to 1886, Freud had been so impressed that he'd translated Charcot's lectures into German and returned eagerly to Vienna to convince his colleagues of the merits of hypnosis in treating hysteria. But the Viennese medical elite weren't impressed: they believed hypnosis was nothing more than quackery.

In his private practice in Vienna, Freud continued to see hysterics, although none presented as dramatically as those seen he'd seen at the Salpêtrière. He treated them with the 'standard weapons in the neurologist's repertoire: massage, hydro-therapeutics, electricity, and the rest cure'.[51] What sparked the Freudian psychoanalytic theories we know most well today was Freud's friendship with the physician Josef Breuer, and Breuer's treatment of a woman named Bertha Pappenheim, better known to the world as Anna O. The fact it was all based on a lie wasn't revealed for over a century—and by then, Freudian psycho-analysis had made its lasting impact on American psychology.

From 1880 to 1882, Breuer had treated Pappenheim for hysteria following the death of her father. According to Scull, her symptoms were dramatic: 'trance-like states, hallucinations, spasms of coughing, sleeplessness, a refusal to eat or drink, a rigid paralysis of the extremities on the right side of her body, severely disturbed vision, outbreaks of uncontrollable anger, a failure to recognise those around her, and finally a failure of language—first a deterioration of her German, then an inability to speak or comprehend anything but English, her native language remaining unintelligible to her for eighteen months'.[52] Breuer regularly talked with Pappenheim about her symptoms and helped her trace them back to traumatic events in her past. This catharsis, according to Breuer, made each symptom disappear. It was Pappenheim who dubbed this method the 'talking cure'.

Breuer became famous for curing Pappenheim but she wasn't cured at all. She was institutionalised by her family shortly after he stopped treating her[53] and remained ill for years after. She only recovered when her first book was published in 1890. She became a social worker, writer and feminist; translating Mary Wollstonecraft's *Vindication of the Rights of Woman* into German, writing a play called *Women's Rights*, and was the co-founder and director of the Judischer Frauenbund, the League of Jewish Women. 'Rather than continuing her role as the passive hysterical patient, through writing she became one who controlled her own cure,' wrote Elaine Showalter.[54]

In 1889 Freud began using hypnosis and the cathartic talking cure on his female patients. He and Breuer wrote a book called *Studies on Hysteria*, in which they claimed that hysteria was the physical manifestation of repressed memories and that it was a sign of superiority, which just so happened to be very good for business.

By the time their book was released in 1895, however, Freud and Breuer had fallen out. Breuer stopped treating hysterics, and Freud came to the conclusion that what he'd believed was permanent relief from hypnosis and the talking cure was in fact only temporary. He devoted his energy to trying to decipher the psychological aspect of hysteria from the physiological, something no one had been able to convincingly unpick. He continued to believe repressed memories were at fault and spent time working out how to get his patients to remember their original trauma. He tried concentration and hypnosis, and then free association: simply getting the patient to speak of whatever came to mind. While he was coming to see hysteria as a psychological condition, he argued its impact was every bit of an illness as pathological disease.

In 1895, he believed hysteria was the result of childhood sexual abuse. But just a year later, after his father died and he suffered from hysteria-like complaints himself, he concluded that these memories of abuse were just sexual fantasies—he couldn't believe there were as many paedophiles as he had patients and, besides, his treatments weren't working.

Freud was depressed, riven with self-doubt, obsessively preoccupied with death, and had regular gastric upsets and heart problems. According to Scull: 'By analysing himself and his dreams, and setting those experiences alongside what he learned from other patients, he moved towards a wholly psychological account of the origins of hysteria.'[55] It took Freud a decade to develop the theory in full; in 1905, he laid it out in *Three Essays on the Theory of Sexuality*.

Some of Freud's most disturbing practices can be seen in his treatment of a patient he called Dora, whose real name was Ida Bauer. She was brought to Freud by her father with a few hysteric symptoms: depression, headaches and a nervous cough.[56] She was frustrated by the confined life she was expected to live and wanted to pursue further education. And she was the product of a traumatic family history: a family friend, Herr K, had repeatedly attempted to seduce her when she was fourteen; after her complaints to her parents went unheeded, Dora felt she'd been 'handed over to Herr K' for his complicity in the affair Dora's father was having with Herr K's wife.[57] Rather than blame Dora's trauma on the sexual assault, along with the betrayal she must have felt towards her parents, Freud told Dora that she was attracted to her abuser, that she was in love with her father and with Freud himself, and that the repression of her true wishes was the cause of her illness. Dora broke off the treatment. The psychologist Erik Erikson has written of the case: 'Dora had been traumatised, and Freud retraumatised her.'[58]

While Freud listened to his patients in a way earlier physicians hadn't, he didn't trust them as narrators of their experiences. The purpose of his psychoanalysis was to reconstruct their lives and for them to accept his reconstruction. Unable to shrug off Victorian ideas of female deviance, he believed gastric upsets associated with hysteria were a result of masturbation. He saw few hysterics after Dora and concentrated on other neuroses, but his work defined the treatment of female psychological torment for generations to come.

Twentieth century to today

In the early twentieth century, hysteria became closely linked to feminism and the suffrage movement. Feminism itself was considered a form of hysteria, but this diagnosis all but died out after World War I.

Many veterans returned from the war with symptoms of hysteria. In medicine's eternal quest to redefine male hysteria as a separate illness, their condition was called shell shock after World War I, then it became Gulf War syndrome in the 1990s, and today it's most commonly understood as post-traumatic stress disorder (PTSD). Not to say that the redefinition made the diagnosis respectable. In the early twentieth century, the shame of the diagnosis was severe: men who suffered from shell shock were considered weak and defective, 'cowardly malingerers shirking their duty',[59] and if it's not quite as blatant today, the stigma surrounding veterans' PTSD still exists inside and outside the military.

Scull, Rousseau, Showalter and Ussher argue that while hysteria has disappeared from the language of medical diagnosis, it has been renamed as other—still gendered—illnesses, now mostly understood to be psychological. During the twentieth century, hysteria manifested in diagnoses from the psychiatrist's bible, the *Diagnostic and Statistical Manual of Mental Disorders*, such as dissociative disorder (conversion type), somatisation disorder, psychogenic pain disorder, Briquet's syndrome, histrionic personality disorder, undifferentiated somatoform disorder, factitious disorder, and anxieties of all kinds. Women were still institutionalised in mental facilities at much higher rates than men throughout the twentieth century.

In her 2011 book *The Madness of Women*, Jane Ussher argues that in the 21st century hysteria has been redefined as madness in women, specifically in diagnoses of depression, PTSD and borderline personality disorder, which all substantially favour women. Ussher says most of these diagnoses pathologise the reasonable responses of women to their life circumstances, particularly in cases where they've suffered sexual abuse or trauma. In pathologising these responses, she argues, as a society we ignore the conditions that create the trauma: the objectification and sexualisation of women, which leads to the normalisation of sexual abuse, assault, rape and other violence against women.

Hysteria has at times been interpreted by feminists as the ultimate act of protest against the conditions of an era. I think Ussher's right, but I would go further to say that the social conditions of living in a patriarchal society are causing these modern versions of hysteria, and in that sense, nothing much has changed. But we should never lose sight of the fact that female hysterics of the past must have had illnesses that were unknown by medical science at the time. Women then, as now, were in genuine pain and distress, and medicine couldn't help them.

The ways in which hysteria has historically been diagnosed and treated have infected medical beliefs about women's health to this day. The distrust of women's narration of their lives survives in medical practice. Just like hysteria was applied as a diagnosis to anything the physician didn't understand,[60] today when women and others with female reproductive systems present with illnesses that defy current understandings of the body, they're diagnosed with medically unexplained symptoms, depression, other mental illnesses or simply disbelieved.

As I see it, there are two parts to the puzzle of hysteria's survival in the 21st century. The first involves the set of patients with diagnosable diseases. Many patients diagnosed with hysteria in centuries past would have had physical diseases we'd recognise today as epilepsy, anaemia, arthritis, multiple sclerosis, brain tumours, anorexia nervosa, endometriosis, migraine, chronic fatigue syndrome, fibromyalgia, as well as other chronic pain conditions and autoimmune diseases. It would seem on the surface good that we now recognise these conditions, right? Well, yes, many women with these conditions undoubtedly fare better today than they would have in the past—but many of these conditions are beset by extensive delays in diagnosis, showing that women are still being written off as hysterical before having their symptoms adequately investigated. Even *after* diagnosis, many patients are still treated by medical professionals as hysterical. We can see it in the way doctors and medical literature talk about some of these conditions, and the people who suffer from them, and in how little research funding has been allocated to discovering more about them.

The second piece of the puzzle involves the set of patients diagnosed with any of the mental health diagnoses widely acknowledged as modern versions of hysteria—depression, anxiety, PTSD, borderline personality disorder. These conditions often cause immense suffering in the patient and medicine continues to struggle with appropriate and adequate treatments. The woman is still blamed for her anguish, her pain and her distress. She is still hysterical.

Rousseau wrote that the most revelatory dimensions of hysteria remain 'its basis in gender and social class power and control'.[61] In that case, he argues, hysteria will never disappear because it essentially reinvents itself to reflect the cultures it imitates.

Once again, the world is undergoing vast and speedy changes, with people's lives barely comparable to those even a generation ago. Oppressive social conditions are creating stress and illness in women, minorities and people of low socio-economic backgrounds. Stress, anxiety, depression and chronic pain are endemic. Just as Cheyne and Beard declared hysteria a disease of industrialisation and accomplishment, so too depression, anxiety and chronic illness are put down as responses to rapid globalisation and technological advance today.

The theory is so prevalent, it shows up in popular culture, so offhand as to appear almost callous. In Sally Rooney's *Conversations with Friends* (which incidentally includes the best description of endometriosis pain I've ever read), the main character, Frances, responds to her boyfriend revealing he has severe depression with the statement, 'Bobbi thinks depression is a humane response to the conditions of late capitalism.'[62]

And here hysteria lurks—imitating the culture of its time.

CHAPTER 4

Neither Madonna nor whore: rethinking female sexuality

A reading of the history of hysteria makes it abundantly clear how a woman's health has been inextricably linked to her sexuality. Masturbation, too much sex, not enough sex, too much desire for sex and even just the thought of sex have all, at different points in history, been claimed to be causes of illness. In ancient Western society it was a voracious womb wandering lustfully through the body in search of nourishment, and later it was simply female sexual appetite that became suspect and pathologised, needing to be contained for the good of society. But a woman is also required to have sex in order to reproduce and to satisfy her male partner; this is the conundrum a woman still faces today.

Dr Kate Young, a Monash University public health researcher, has summed up the dilemma: 'Medical texts have historically constructed women's sexuality as volatile and in need of control; uncontrolled, it would lure men from their intellectual pursuits and distract women from their assigned reproductive role. However, if women are to fulfil this reproductive role, it is necessary for them to engage in (penis-vaginal) sex with men. Thus, women are expected to endure but not enjoy sex, and the physical ability to do so became medically pathologised while little to no consideration was given to their sexual pleasure.'[1]

The effects of these beliefs echo through the ages. As women, shame around our sexuality is often felt so deeply that we're unable to use the correct words for our anatomy. Our education about our bodies is incomplete, and the silence around menstruation means it too becomes shameful and linked to sex.

All of this is disastrous for our understanding of our bodies, our health, our pleasure, our desire, our happiness and our relationships. But it's an effective means for men to retain control over us.

As Barbara Ehrenreich and Deirdre English have argued, medicine didn't become the primary enforcer of sexism in our society because doctors are somehow inherently sexist—it took over from religion because it was more effective.[2] Today, a woman's access to her own reproductive rights is controlled by doctors. If she wants to prevent, terminate or pursue a pregnancy, she must see a doctor, most likely several, even when she isn't sick, and even though medical intervention is necessary in some but not all reproductive medicine.

That's not to say religion no longer plays a role in upholding the sexist structures that govern Western society. A vast majority of cultures worldwide still have one belief in common: women should be essentially chaste and subject to a man, and repress their sexuality outside of his bedroom. A sexually liberated women is considered a threat so severe, any transgression must be punished, sometimes ruthlessly.

In *Down Girl: The logic of misogyny*, Cornell University professor of philosophy Kate Manne argues that misogyny is not about an individual man hating all women but about social power relations. Misogyny can be seen in how society polices women in order to ensure they fulfil their socially prescribed gendered roles and punishes those who don't. The test of misogyny can't, then, be whether a man loves his mother, wife or daughters—of course a man will love his wife, mother or daughters if they have provided him with 'the nurturing, comfort, care,' and/or the 'sexual, emotional and reproductive labor'[3] that society tells him he is entitled to. The real test of misogyny is in how the man responds to women who refuse to offer him those resources, and especially those women who may be competing with him for a position traditionally held to be the domain of man. This would help explain why female writers, actors, gamers and politicians are so severely trolled online—out of all proportion to men who hold similar views.

It's in this way that secular Western cultures have largely maintained the religious tradition of repressing women's sexuality. Of course there are exceptions, and things are changing (slowly), but the use of shame in Western cultures to enforce adherence to an idealised femininity is still extremely effective. Most Western women still learn to police their behaviour, go to extreme lengths in personal grooming in order to be seen as attractive, and remain largely subservient to the sexual desires of men. And if they are the victims of sexual harassment or assault, they learn to internalise the shame.

The sexual revolution of the 1960s and 70s has been hailed as a turning point in Western civilisation. The contraceptive pill gave women more sexual freedom than their mothers, and many women—myself included—have benefited from this. But the recent revelations of widespread sexual assault and harassment in Hollywood, Westminster, Washington and Silicon Valley—and surely many other industries, yet to be uncovered in such spectacular style—reveal the truth of the sexual revolution: that it freed men to feel comfortable with their fantasies of sexual dominance without uprooting the culture that shames women and people of all genders in lower social classes both for enjoying sex and for speaking out about sexual violence. It's probably worth noting that a factor in how the #MeToo revelations have played in the media is down to how Western systems of justice have failed to adequately deal with the perpetrators of sexual misconduct—both that committed against girls and women, and also against boys and men.

Hugh Hefner's *Playboy* empire, founded in the early 1950s, was lauded by many people as liberating, but I believe it was only really liberating for men. Writing in *The Guardian* following Hefner's death and the first sexual harassment claims against Harvey Weinstein, the American author Rebecca Solnit said that Hefner and his magazines 'insisted that women were for men to use if they met a narrow definition of attractiveness, and to mock or ignore if they were not. While often portrayed as part of the sexual revolution, the magazine and Hefner were instead part of the counter-revolution, figuring out how to perpetuate women's subordination and men's power in a changing era.'[4]

At the core of a lot of sexual violence against women is the belief that they should be passive objects of active male desire. Women are still vilified as being 'sluts' when they engage in casual sexual relationships and still questioned on witness stands about what they were wearing while being raped, and any woman with a sexual history beyond serial monogamy is assumed to be 'asking for it' when she's sexually assaulted.

These days, early exposure to extreme forms of pornography that are essentially degrading to girls and women is harming young people and influencing their behaviour in relationships. And from a casual consumption of current pop culture, you wouldn't know that women enjoy sex as much as men: in too many films and TV shows, songs, books and pornography, sex is something men desire and women relinquish. Too often in pop culture, sex is an act done *to* a woman rather than *with* a woman, and this is highlighted in the wide acceptance that heterosexual sex is over when a man ejaculates.

There are some exceptions but they're few and far between, and they often lack inclusivity. Sure, TV shows like Lena Dunham's *Girls* and Phoebe Waller-Bridge's *Fleabag* show young women desiring and enjoying—as well as *not* enjoying—sex, but all the main characters are of a certain class and colour. Sexuality is steeped in racist prejudice—think of all the demeaning tropes about virile black men and sexualised black women. The British writer and broadcaster Afua Hirsch uses a striking example in her book, *Brit(ish)*, of how Maria

121

Sharapova's sexuality is treated compared to Venus and Serena Williams': 'a white woman's sexuality is cheeky, fun and tasteful; a black woman's offensive, off-putting and indecent'.[5] Hirsch quotes from a 2015 *Daily Mail* article by Alison Boshoff to illustrate her point: '[Serena] Williams, 33, is the more physically powerful, with a ferocious temper and the mindset of a battling champion. However, she cannot compete with Sharapova's media-friendly combination of blonde Siberian beauty.'

Asian women are also subject to dangerous sexual stereotypes. While it has been centuries in the making—see the sexualised images of Japanese geisha in the Victorian era or watch the *Thief of Baghdad* (1924) for how it was once applied to veiled Middle Eastern women—today the fetishisation of Asian women by white men has become normalised in Western culture. As the comedian Kristina Wong wrote: 'White guys with Asian fetishes used to be easy to spot—pathetic social pariahs planning their sex tour vacations to Thailand, creeping around Japanese language classes. Now, Asiaphiles are attractive tattooed hipsters that possess fantastic social skills, and we meet them through friends of friends.'

In an article for *Bitch Media* outlining the history of the Asian woman fetish by white men, Patricia Park writes that the 'perception of sexualized Asian women was informed by a long tradition of the Western male writing', from Puccini's *Madama Butterfly* to the 1989 musical *Miss Saigon*. But perhaps no better popular culture reference sums it up than the scene from Stanley Kubrick's film, *Full Metal Jacket*, in which a Vietnamese female sex worker says, 'Me so horny. Me love you long time. Me sucky sucky.'[6]

The Asian woman is expected to be both submissive and hypersexual, the ultimate representation of femininity—providing care, nurture, support, sex and emotional and reproductive labour to a dominant white man. But this fetish-isation has perilous real-life consequences: up to 55 per cent of Asian women experience sexual or physical violence by an intimate partner in the United States.[7]

SEXUALITY

From the moment she's old enough to understand, almost every girl is taught that it's her role to be a pleasure giver—after all, what does pleasure have to do with herself?

In *Down Girl*, Manne explains how society raises *human beings*, 'white men who are otherwise privileged in most if not all major respects', and *human givers*, 'a woman who is held to owe many if not most of her distinctively human capacities to a suitable boy or man, ideally, and his children as applicable'.[8] From the youngest possible age, girls are trained to *give* their full humanity: 'A giver is then obligated to offer love, sex, attention, affection, and admiration, as well as other forms of emotional, social, reproductive, and caregiving labor', writes Manne. Meanwhile, boys are raised to express their full humanity, to be competitive, inquisitive, autonomous, to do whatever it takes to be fulfilled—they are human beings.[9] Manne's book is one that Emily Nagoski—an American author, sex educator and former Kinsey Institute researcher—tells me that she can't stop talking about. 'So,' she says, 'if we raise our children within this dichotomy of human givers and human beings, then of course by the time they get to a place where they're having sex with each other, who's going to have sexual pleasure? Who's going to do the giving? And who's going to do the receiving? There is a really straight-forward narrative in place for them already—that narrative is reinforced by all of the porn they watch, it's reinforced by everything their parents are talking to them about. And it's reinforced by the actual experiences that they have.'

Likewise, in *The Madness of Women*, Jane Ussher explains that because 'women are taught to believe that they are not loved for who they are, but for how well they meet the needs of others',[10] they learn to silence their desires and feelings. The widespread cultural standards imposed on women of ideal femininity also leave many women in a constant state of self-judgement, 'leading to feelings of worthlessness and hopelessness'.[11]

These cultural messages are mixed in with those received at school, home and possibly church, that sex is dirty, disgusting and dangerous—but also something a woman should give to a man she loves, and if she's not good at it no one will love her. Confusing, right? And it's not just confusing to women.

Many men are afflicted with the Madonna–whore complex. They want to sleep with a woman who's sexually exciting and adventurous, who knows how to give pleasure; they also want their wife to be demure, pure and chaste. Knowing this, women are left either trying to be both or choosing to be the eternal mistress or the wife whose primary duties are to raise children, stay silent about her husband's affairs and provide sex to make him happy. Neither of these options sounds ideal, does it? But this dichotomy has persisted to the present day for many women around the world.

Sexuality has, until very recently, always been viewed through the male prism. In her seminal book *Come as You Are:*

The surprising new science that will transform your sex life, Emily Nagoski wrote: 'For a long, long time in Western science and medicine, women's sexuality was viewed as Men's Sexuality Lite—basically the same but not quite as good.'[12] In general, when women have experienced sexual desire, pleasure or arousal in different ways to men, this has been seen as just another example of women's deficiency. It's hard to overplay the importance of Nagoski's book in exposing female sexuality for its full, rich and, yes, pleasurable existence. She turns almost everything we thought we knew about sex on its head.

When I ask Nagoski why only 62 per cent of women having sex with men compared to 86 per cent of men having sex with women say they orgasm during sex (the figure rises to 75 per cent for women having sex with women), she tells me the only people interested in the orgasm gap are journalists. 'In fact, using the standard of orgasm is itself patriarchal,' she informs me. 'We are very used to measuring women's sexual wellbeing in terms of men's sexuality. And we assume that the ways in which women are different from men must be the ways in which women are inferior or broken or diseased when in fact it might be that women are just different.'

While skyping with Nagoski, I tell her how often I've thought about her contention that stress, mood, trust and body image are all central to a woman's sexual wellbeing. I've always imagined sexual wellbeing as being intricately tied to a woman's physical and mental health, her work/life burden and, ultimately, her place in society. Nagoski says, 'Strangely or not, the best predictor of a woman's sexual wellbeing is her overall wellbeing, which is why those issues—stress, mood, relationships—are not peripheral, it's because they're determining factors in whether or not she's experiencing whatever you want to call sexual wellbeing.'

While sexual wellbeing can't be summarised neatly here— you'll have to read Nagoski's book for that—she says the key to understanding what 'sexuality' means is to understand what's 'normal' and what's 'pleasurable'. 'For me, there are only two things that are not normal. One is pain. It is not normal to experience pain with sex—unwanted pain, I should say. If you are being spanked and you love that, great. If you're experiencing genital pain with intercourse, that's not normal, that's a medical condition, you can find a physical therapist who can help you with it. A lot of sexual pain is treatable, we now know. The only other thing that doesn't count as normal is lack of consent.'

In January 2018, during the #MeToo movement, Babe.net published a woman's account of a difficult and unpleasant date with the American comedian Aziz Ansari which recounted how Ansari placed incredible sexual pressure on the young woman and failed to respond to her verbal and non-verbal cues that she didn't want to have sex with him.* Lili Loofbourow responded with an essay in *The Week*, 'The Female Price of Male Pleasure',[13] which is one of the most affecting pieces of writing I've ever read. She starts by giving an explanation to all the people around the world asking why-oh-why did the young woman not leave the date with Ansari the minute she started to feel uncomfortable: 'Women are enculturated to be uncomfortable most of the time. And to ignore their discomfort.'

★   Ansari issued a statement after the article was published saying that he felt the sexual activity was 'by all indications completely consensual. [I]t was true that everything did seem OK to me, so when I heard that it was not the case for her, I was surprised and concerned.'

Loofbourow's essay then goes deeper, exploring the extraordinary pain women suffer in order to provide men with pleasure. And they mostly suffer it in silence. According to Loofbourow, the problem with the men-have-biological-needs argument—that it's in men's nature to chase women and be dominant in the sack—isn't just that it is scientific garbage. 'The real problem isn't that we—as a culture—don't sufficiently consider men's biological reality. The problem is rather that theirs is literally *the only biological reality* we ever bother to consider.' It's true that we know more about male biology than female biology. We know more about male sexuality; we know more about male health—this is all related.

'Research shows that 30 per cent of women report pain during vaginal sex, 72 per cent report pain during anal sex, and "large proportions" don't tell their partners when sex hurts,' Loofbourow says. She quotes Professor Debby Herbenick from the Indiana University School of Public Health, who is an expert on human sexuality, as saying: 'When it comes to "good sex" . . . women often mean without pain, men often mean they had orgasms.'[14]

The stats back up the story: *PubMed* has 393 clinical trials studying dyspareunia, the medical term for pain during sexual intercourse. There are ten clinical trials studying vaginismus and 43 for vulvodynia. How many for erectile dysfunction—which, as Loofbourow says, 'while lamentable, is not painful'? One thousand nine hundred and fifty-four. 'That's right: *PubMed* has almost five times as many clinical trials on male sexual pleasure as it has on female sexual pain. And why? Because we live in a culture that sees female pain as normal and male pleasure as a right.'[15]

To understand the full picture of women's sexuality, it's essential to realise that pleasure, arousal, desire and consent are separate elements—and they aren't always related. Out of the four, pleasure is probably the aspect we know least about.

Clinical sexologist and relationships counsellor Nina Booysen tells me that often the women she sees who are struggling with desire are those who never learnt to self-pleasure as girls. For one reason or another, they got the message that masturbation was dirty, that they had no right to pleasure. 'For women to learn to self-pleasure and self-serve is so, so important to be able to sustain the desire and their sexuality later on in life,' she says. 'I do believe that women don't really invest in themselves as sexual beings.'

Changing the habits of a lifetime can be hard. That's why Booysen tells her clients to start with the simplest pleasures: savouring a bite of chocolate, feeling the shower's water wash over your skin—a kind of mindfulness of pleasant sensory experiences. The team at OMGYes has gone a step further, uploading video demonstrations of the most common techniques women use to masturbate.

OMGYes points out that there's never been any large-scale research done on female sexual pleasure, so they teamed up with Indiana University and the Kinsey Institute, one of the world's leading authorities on human sexuality, to talk to more than 2000 women, aged eighteen to 95, about the techniques they used to reach orgasm. They found that lots of these techniques were similar but there were no words yet to describe them. 'One of the casualties of the taboo around women's pleasure is that there aren't words for the important ways touch can vary,' says OMGYes on its website. 'There are vague, clinical words like stimulate and vague, pop-culture words like fingering and rubbing. This lack of language makes it far harder to explore and find new things that work. Imagine trying a new recipe, but none of the ingredients or measurements have names. Or ordering from a menu but all of the dishes are called the same thing.'[16]

According to OMGYes's research, women who are able to talk specifically about what makes sex more pleasurable for them are eight times more likely to be happier in their relationships. Couples who keep exploring new ways to increase pleasure are five times more likely to be happier in their relationships and twelve times more likely to be sexually satisfied.

Nagoski acknowledges that the science on female sexual pleasure is a little behind, but she's adamant most women do experience sexual pleasure when the context is right. 'And that context is important,' she says. She talks me through some lab testing on rats that shows how one type of sensation can lead to different—positive or negative—reactions depending on the rat's environment. When researchers zapped the front of a part of the brain called the nucleus accumbens, the rat approached with curiosity; when they zapped the back of the nucleus accumbens, it responded in a threatened manner called defensive tread and bury. However, in a peaceful 'home environment, the same zap to the back of the nucleus accumbens was greeted with the same curious, exploratory behaviour as when the front was zapped'.

What does this mean for humans? 'If you can imagine a context where you're already in a super flirty playful fun state of mind, feeling really turned on already and your partner tickles you and that can feel good and lead to other things. But if you're in the middle of trying to get the kids out the door to go to school and your partner tickles you, or if you're pissed off at your partner, how does that feel when they tickle you? Kind of like you want to punch them in the face, a little bit,' she tells me.

'And nothing has changed about the sensation, it's the same person touching you in the same way but because the context is different your brain interprets that sensation totally differently. So pleasure is not a simple, "I like to be touched in this particular way", or "I like to be touched in this particular part of my body", it's "I like to be touched when I'm in a particular state of mind, when the world is treating me in a particular way".

'Which is a much bigger ask, it's a heavier lift than, "touch me on my neck, lightly".'

Pleasure isn't the same thing as arousal, which isn't the same as desire. So what are the differences between them, and why are these important to understand? Well, again, I encourage anyone who's ever felt sexually inadequate or somehow deficient to read *Come as You Are*. But when I speak to her, Nagoski kindly sums it up: 'Arousal is the process of your body responding to a sexually relevant stimulus. Sexual pleasure is your body experiencing that sexually relevant stimulus in the right context. Desire is what happens when your body experiences a sexually relevant stimulus in the right context and it activates a desire for more.'

And then there's consent. A person can want something and it can feel good, but they may still not want to go further. Our bodies can show outward signs of arousal—for example, a vagina may become lubricated, or a person may even orgasm—in a context where it's not pleasurable and not wanted. At any point during a sexual encounter, however someone's body is responding, if they say 'no' this should be respected—but sometimes it isn't. Nagoski talks about how this can happen in relationships. 'If they're having sex with a partner who's pushing them to do things that they don't want to do, if their body's responding, their partner will use that genital response as kind of a weapon against their partner, and say, "well your body's responding, so your body's saying yes even if you're saying no". What? No, arousal and pleasure are not the same thing. And it's certainly not consent.'

It can also work the other way: a woman may be very turned on and want to continue with sexual intercourse but her vagina and vulva may be dry, not lubricated, which her male partner takes to believe she's not enjoying it, even though she tells him she is. This seemingly contradictory response is actually completely normal and can happen to anyone, no matter what genitals they have.

Officially, both of these situations are called arousal non-concordance, and two decades of research on this phenomenon has shown again and again how prevalent it is. The take-out? The only way you can tell if somebody is experiencing pleasure and wants to continue is to ask, listen and believe the answer.

Desire is another complicated factor in human sexuality that has a cultural meaning quite removed from people's lived experience. To understand desire, it helps to get acquainted with the dual control model, a concept developed by researchers Erick Janssen and John Bancroft at the Kinsey Institute in the 1990s but widely popularised by Nagoski. In her book, she describes this model as the 'why' and 'how' of human sexuality; she puts it simply: 'Your sexual brain has an "accelerator" that responds to sexual stimulation, but it also has "brakes" which respond to all the very good reasons not to be turned on right now.'[17]

The sexual accelerator, she writes, 'responds to "sexually relevant" stimulation—anything you see, hear, smell, touch, taste, or imagine that your brain has learned to associate with sexual arousal.'

The brain's sexual brakes, on the other hand, 'respond to "potential threats"—anything you see, hear, smell, touch, taste or imagine that your brain interprets as a good reason not to be turned on right now. These can be anything from STDs and unwanted pregnancy to relationship issues or social reputation.'

Importantly, she adds: 'There's virtually no "innate" sexually relevant stimulus or threat; our accelerators and brakes learn when to respond through experience. And that learning process is different for males and females.'[18]

Booysen finds this concept incredibly helpful in her practice. She says we often forget that the brain is our biggest sex organ; we need to be able to recognise—and perhaps savour—when we see, hear or notice something that gives us that 'little ping of horniness'. Booysen adds: 'What women with low desire tend to do is that they shut that off so quickly. They push it away so quickly, the brakes come on so hard, and eventually they don't even realise they're doing it.'

Nagoski agrees that often when people are struggling with sexual desire and arousal, it's because there's too much stimulation to the brake. 'Usually when you're struggling with your sexuality . . . it has nothing to do with your sexuality itself,' she says. 'A lot of it has to do with the other stuff in your life. Like you're feeling stressed out and exhausted or not really great about body image stuff these days or not feeling really great in your relationship. Those are really important factors that can't be fixed by doing something to your sexuality.'

In other words, no amount of sex toys or role-playing will fix this issue—it's like driving a car with the handbrake on, Nagoski says. It's important to learn what's leading the brake to turn on and how to separate desire from pleasure. Most people do want pleasure in their lives; they do want sexual intimacy with their partners. Yet for those who've experienced sexual trauma, any sex-related stimulus may mean they end up hitting the brakes hard every time they hit the accelerator. Their brain learns, explains Nagoski, that any sexual stimulus is a threat and treats it like a life-or-death situation. 'This is profoundly subconscious, it's not a deliberate choice,' Nagoski tells me, then adds the good news: the experience of arousal can be decoupled from the feeling of threat or fear. 'It takes time and patience and self-compassion but people heal from sexual trauma all the time.'

Everyone can be affected by cultural norms around sex, and about half of the clients Booysen sees in Darwin are cisgender men experiencing a lack of desire. Nagoski points to US statistics: in half the heterosexual couples seeking sex therapy because of a lack of desire, the man is the partner with this issue. So the idea that *all* men want sex *all* the time simply isn't true.

But the widespread belief in this comes from somewhere, right? In *Come as You Are*, Nagoski explains different desire styles. Spontaneous desire is what we tend to associate with men: a person can think about and want sex spontaneously, just walking down the street, all the time. It's a 'totally normal way to experience desire', Nagoski tells me. But there's also what researchers call responsive desire, and it emerges in response to pleasure. It can work like this: I'm sitting on the sofa with a glass of wine, totally relaxed, and my partner starts touching me in a way that feels very pleasurable—here my desire kicks in. This is more typically experienced by women than men but it's by no means a gender-based dichotomy. In fact, Nagoski recalls, 'When I wrote an op-ed in the *New York Times* about [responsive desire], I actually got more emails from men than women, saying thank you, this language describes what I have been experiencing. And it's not a pathology, it's normal.'

Nagoski says: 'The more we increase the conversation around the diversity of women's sexual experiences, the more space we make for the diversity of men's sexual experiences too.' This serves as a reminder that culture does change and has changed—in many parts of the world, women are experiencing greater sexual freedom than in the previous generation. 'In my own lifetime I can feel the difference that has happened,' Nagoski says. 'I started doing work around sexual violence prevention around 1996. And just last year the MeToo movement happened, and it felt like the work I had been doing for two decades had finally cracked something open.

'And now not only are we talking about women's basic bodily autonomy, we're even beginning to talk about masculinity, and the ways that it is toxic to men and the ways that what patriarchy says masculinity has to be is the actual cause of men perpetrating violence. Of men believing that women don't have a right to say no, of men's sexual entitlement. That we stop talking about bad apples and the individual bad people, certainly there are those serial perpetrators who just totally feel like they're allowed to do anything that they want to someone else's body, but most guys are nice guys. And are just now under the avalanche of stories that are being shared about a combination of a lack of consent and a lack of pleasure—they're being forced to look at the assumptions they've been making about their bodies and their partners'. Which is good. It's uncomfortable for everybody but it creates a space where we can say: what can we change for women and men in order to make sex better for both of them.'

For centuries, men have been taught to chase and women to play hard to get. This is why the Aziz Ansari case was one of the most instructive for me. Ansari committed no crime but he displayed an alarming lack of sensitivity and insight into issues of consent for a bloke who literally wrote the book on 'modern romance'.[19] The public conversation that started after the Ansari story broke has helped to challenge the bad apple theory: that only terrible men hurt women. It's also brought into the spotlight the harmful idea that men have to chase and women have to say no until finally relenting. Again, this is the Madonna–whore complex playing out—if a woman does say no at first and then relents, it allows the man to believe she's a good girl, worthy of being his wife, and his charm and suave moves have made her give in; if she says yes too readily, she's the whore who won't get a phone call in the morning.

If #MeToo achieves anything, I hope it's the death of the idea that it's a pure biological force that men need to, or should be the ones to, chase women and that it's natural and right for women to play hard to get.

Angela Saini's book *Inferior* should play a huge role in debunking this myth. In it, she recounts in fascinating detail the battle of the sexes in evolutionary biology. On one hand, we have mostly male researchers—starting with Charles Darwin and his 1871 book *The Descent of Man, and Selection in Relation to Sex* and moving on to research done in 1948 on fruit flies—who have theorised that men are promiscuous and undiscriminating and that women are highly discriminating and sexually passive. Some of the work based on fruit flies became so famous that it was used in a 1998 article for the *New Yorker* titled 'Boys will be boys: An evolutionary explanation for Presidents behaving badly', by the cognitive psychologist Steven Pinker to excuse Bill Clinton's affair with Monica Lewinsky.[20]

On the other hand, we have many female scientists, and male scientists as well, who have accumulated countless studies showing that these assumptions just aren't true across all species. Saini shows how research in langur monkeys, primates, birds, small-mouth salamanders, bush crickets, yellow-pine chipmunks, prairie dogs and meal-worm beetles have disproved the neat theory on female monogamy.

It was also debunked in humans, from anthropological studies on the Himba tribe in Namibia, the matriarchal Mosuo of China, some isolated South American societies, as well as in studies tracking reproductive success in Finland, Iran, Brazil and Mali.

Could it be—as Brooke Scelza, the behavioural ecologist who studied the Himba tribe, told Saini—that the rules about how women and men behave in relationships have more to do with society than with biology? And Saini raises the most interesting question of all: if females are naturally chaste and coy, why do males go to such extraordinary lengths to keep them faithful?

SEX AS A METHOD OF CONTROL
Throughout history, men have gone to incredible lengths to ensure women remain chaste, virgins until they're married

and faithful to their husbands. The list of horrific punishments inflicted on women who fail to act out their supposedly passive and monogamous natures is long.

Despite being illegal in most countries today, women are still murdered by their families in so-called honour killings for committing adultery or having sex before marriage, among other reasons. Stoning remains a punishment for women who have affairs in Saudi Arabia, Sudan, Iran, Yemen, Somalia, parts of Nigeria and Indonesia; while it's outlawed in Pakistan and Afghanistan, it still takes place. In 2015, footage emerged online of the stoning of a nineteen-year-old woman accused of adultery in Taliban-controlled Afghanistan. CNN described it like this: 'The men surround the woman as she stands in a hole dug into the stony ground, only her head pokes above the surface. Then they begin to pick up rocks and hurl them at her again and again from close range. Her agonised cries grow louder as the barrage of stones intensifies.'[21]

Two other examples often used as evidence of patriarchal control over women are Chinese foot binding and the African tradition of female genital mutilation.

The bandaging of women's feet to restrict their growth and change their shape was practised in China from the tenth to the twentieth centuries; it was particularly prevalent among upper-class women, who were more able to be spared from work and more easily restricted to the home. Bound feet were considered a sign of beauty and class—the ultimate fashion statement. But the practice was equally a measure of social control: these women, who could barely walk and could never run away, were literally hobbled to live dependent on their husband and family.

In female genital mutilation, a girl's external clitoris is removed to hobble her desire. If a woman doesn't enjoy sex, the theory behind it goes, she's very unlikely to leave her husband for another man. The UN estimates at least 200 million women and girls alive today have undergone female genital mutilation in the 30 countries on which it has data.[22] In most of these countries, the majority of girls were cut before age five. With migration, female genital mutilation is now a problem in countries such as the US, UK and Australia.

Sexual domination is another method of patriarchal control. Sex and power are intricately linked—we know that rape and sexual assault and even sexual harassment aren't about sex and attraction but about control. It's always been like this.

In discussing the ways in which homosexuality has been pathologised as a disease, Mike McRae wrote in *Unwell*, 'One possibility is that sex among social animals like us isn't just about pleasure and reproduction. It's about reinforcing a social order. Think of it as a political exchange, a way to strengthen bonds with those close to us. As such, it's also a firm statement about who we are as a group. As the glue that binds us, how we have sex can form the basis of sorting "us" from "them".'[23] This also makes sense of why men's sexual misconduct towards women is so prevalent: it's partly a way for men to reinforce their superiority over women, especially effective when there are few or no repercussions or consequences for the action, and to form bonds with their peers. The Belgian psychotherapist and author Esther Perel told the Pleasure Mechanics podcast that sex and power have been so culturally entangled that some men feel entitled to 'sexual access to women, especially women of lower social status';

she said these men 'claimed it as a job benefit' and never think they'll be held accountable.[24]

The statistics are stark. More than a third of women (35 per cent) globally have experienced physical or sexual violence in their lives.[25] Approximately 15 million girls between the ages of fifteen and nineteen have been sexually assaulted (forced into sexual intercourse or other sexual acts).[26] Between 10 and 69 per cent of women are physically assaulted by an intimate male partner.[27] In Australia, 39 per cent of women and 26 per cent of men have been sexually harassed at work in the past five years—four out of five harassers were men.[28] In the United States, one in six women has been the victim of an attempted or completed rape.[29] In Egypt, 99 per cent of women say they've been sexually harassed.[30] Half of transgender people in the US have been sexually abused. Forty-four per cent of American lesbians and 61 per cent of American bisexual women experience rape, physical violence, or stalking by an intimate partner.[31]

When class and race intersect with gender, the situation is even worse. The abuse and assault of women of colour has been a fundamental aspect of colonisation everywhere it took place. Female slaves in the United States were raped and sometimes taken as concubines by their white owners; obviously it was very hard for them to fight back, but instead of eliciting sympathy this fuelled ideas among white people that African women were hypersexual and lustful. A similar fate befell the Indigenous women of Australia and many other women of colour around the world.

In Australia today, Indigenous women are 32 times more likely to be hospitalised due to family violence than non-Indigenous women. One in seven Indigenous women has experienced physical violence in the past year.[32] In the UK, black and minority ethnic (BME) women suffer from higher levels of domestic homicide, honour killings and abuse-driven suicide than white women. The policy and research consultant Hannana Siddiqui has noted the current challenges: 'The rise of religious fundamentalism or ultra conservative forces within and outside of minority communities (in all religions and internationally) has increased pressure on BME women to conform to traditional gender roles and strengthened justifications for the use of violence to chasten transgressors.'[33]

These shocking statistics are no accident, argues Jane Ussher, but the direct result of a society that objectifies women: 'The sexual objectification of women occurs on a continuum—ranging from the depiction of girls and women as sexualised objects in the media or in pornography, to the enactment of sexual violence and abuse.'[34]

This highly sexualised society creates a double bind for women: they have to be sexy to be attractive but if they're sexy and abused, it's their fault. Speaking of the historic duty of wives, Esther Perel describes this dilemma:

His duty was to provide, her duty was to please him . . . But that's just one piece. The other piece was that her duty was also to make sure that he doesn't transgress because the body of women has never belonged to women, they belong to society. And women have to deal with their bodies, cover their bodies, you know, restrict themselves in all kinds of ways in order for men not to have their lustful urges take the better of them . . . So women have consistently been

NEITHER MADONNA NOR WHORE

perceived in two directions—uber powerful or degraded . . .
She either is the one that is so powerful that he can't resist
her, therefore if he trespasses it's because of her . . . And on
the other side she has no rights, she's his possession and he
gets to do with her what he wants in return for feeding her,
taking care of her children . . .[35]

As the Australian feminist and former editor-in-chief of *Ms*
magazine Anne Summers argued in her influential 1975 book,
women are expected to be God's police, saying no to sexual
advances and protecting both their own, and society's, morals.
If they don't fulfil this role, they're damned whores.[36]

While white, Western, cisgender women may experience
greater sexual freedom today than was imaginable even a
generation ago—and I count myself among these women—
progress isn't linear. Sexual domination of men over women
continues today, with new forces behind it.

Young people are having less sex than Generation Xers
and Baby Boomers did when they were young—in the US,
the percentage of high school students in years 9 to 12 who
have had sex dropped from 54 to 41 per cent between 1991
and 2015[37]—and the pleasure of girls and women is, in many
cases, being neglected. Research in 2014 that looked at the
sex lives of young people in England found an uncomfortable social setting 'where women's pleasure and desires are
neglected, where painful sex for women is seen as normal
and where there appears to be a real risk of coercion,' one
of the researchers, Cicely Marston, wrote in *The Conversation*. 'Our interviewees described an oppressive environment
where some men compete with each other to have anal sex

with women, even if they expect women to find it painful. Coercion seems to be seen as normal: women reported they were repeatedly asked for anal sex by their male partners, and men's and women's accounts also raise the real possibility of unwanted penetration for young women—who are sometimes put in situations where they are penetrated anally without their explicit consent.'[38]

Nina Booysen says that the extreme pornography young people are now exposed to online is changing sexuality in general, to the detriment of women. 'Porn is shaping the sexual lives and core beliefs of women,' Booysen says. She tells me she has many young male clients who can't maintain an erection while having sex with a male or female partner. 'They're absolutely fine when they're watching porn but when there's a live human being in front of them they can't do it.' She's a strong advocate for better education on the safe use of porn and also on improved education about normal human—especially female—anatomy. 'I've had guys calling me up telling me that their girlfriend's dirty . . . [because] she has a dirty bum. I tell him, that's normal pigmentation, mate, everything you're watching on porn, that's bleached . . . skin.' Bleached anuses, labiaplasty and hairless vulvas have all been normalised by pornography among younger people. But that's not the worst of it, she says. 'Girls are under this huge pressure now to live up to being a porn star, and do things that are degrading and dehumanising and painful to please boys, because if they don't do that—the boys can't function.'

Anita Saldanha, a GP who works in a small rural Australian town, expressed similar concern about young women's rela-tionship to sex and with their own sexuality. Having gone to the local high school to talk about bullying, when she asked if there were any questions the sixteen-year-old girls were eager to talk about sex and contraception. She was shocked they couldn't identify their ovaries or cervix on a diagram, had no idea what a pap smear was for, only a vague idea why they'd all had the HPV vaccine, and the only contraceptives they knew about were condoms and the pill. While they told her they knew it was 'normal' for boys to 'wank', nobody had ever told them it was normal for girls to masturbate and explore their own bodies. When Saldanha asked what sex education they'd had in class, the girls told her their teacher was male and got embarrassed when they said 'vagina' so they didn't ask questions and didn't learn much.

'As far as I can tell, no one has ever taught them how their body works,' Saldanha said to me. 'No one has told them that girls are . . . allowed to enjoy sex, girls are allowed to want to have sex but that sex must be something that you *want* to have.' No lessons on consent were offered at the state high school.

She sees the effects of ignorance in her practice every day, with women who come to her complaining about painful sex but can't identify where it hurts. If she asks whether it's stabbing pain at the vaginal entrance or deeper pain at the cervix, they invariably shrug and make general statements like, 'It hurts down there.'

'They're so divorced from their own being, their own body,' she tells me, adding that she feels they've never been given permission to enjoy or find pleasure in sex.

Dr Clare Fairweather is a GP whose practice focuses on treating pelvic pain and endometriosis patients, many of them young women. She's concerned about the pressure on girls as young as fifteen to perform oral and anal sex, telling me she believes some of them are coerced into sexual acts they find painful. Even though painful intercourse is a side effect of chronic pelvic pain and endo, her young patients continue to engage in sex until it becomes too much to bear. Girls and young women who have sex with boys and young men are today, encouraged by popular culture and porn, normalising painful sexual acts that they don't enjoy because it pleases their male partners. If we don't do more to educate people about their sexual health, the sexual revolution may very well become a counter-revolution.

SEXUAL HEALTH

The World Health Organization defines sexual health as 'a state of physical, emotional, mental and social well-being in relation to sexuality; it is not merely the absence of disease, dysfunction or infirmity. Sexual health requires a positive and respectful approach to sexuality and sexual relationships, as well as the possibility of having pleasurable and safe sexual experiences, free of coercion, discrimination and violence. For sexual health to be attained and maintained, the sexual rights of all persons must be respected, protected and fulfilled.'[39]

For most people, being in a healthy relationship requires sexual wellbeing in both or all partners. Being sexually healthy isn't just about having consensual sex or not having an STI, says Nina Booysen. It's about freedom of choice and freedom of expression. It's about desiring and enjoying sexual intercourse. As Booysen points out 'a lot of women still have coercive sex just to keep their husbands happy—and that's not sexual wellbeing,' she says. In fact, more than four in ten women in

51 countries feel they have no choice but to agree with their husband's sexual demands, according to a 2019 study by the United Nations Population Fund.[40]

Booysen, like Esther Perel, believes sex education should include sexual health, particularly when it comes to healthy relationships. Perel told the Pleasure Mechanics podcast that her hope for the outcome of the #MeToo movement was comprehensive sex education about sexual health:

> we need public health campaigns around sexuality, [to be taught] that sexual health is part of overall health, and part of relational health, and that these things are integrated . . . We need to avoid teaching children that sex is dirty, dangerous, dysfunctional, and creates disease. There's so much to do to create a culture that understands the concept of sexual health and doesn't constantly only focus on sexual problems, sexual crisis, sexual dangers, sexual addiction . . . we need a model of sexual health so we know what we are working towards not only what we're trying to eradicate. Like in all other health. It's one thing to know what not to eat, it's another thing to know what to eat! . . . You also need a model for what is desired, for what will create a different playing field between men and women.[41]

Sexual health is largely left out of most interactions with medical professionals in Western society today. Booysen told me of a cartoon she spotted in a hospital of a doctor sitting with his patient. The doctor is thinking, 'If there's a sexual problem I hope he brings it up.' And the patient is sitting on the bed, thinking, 'I hope he asks.' It's tricky for doctors to talk about sex and sexuality. They're not taught how to have these difficult conversations in medical school, and many fear being seen as offensive if they enquire about sexuality—especially in interactions between male doctors and female patients. Added to this, sexual dysfunction is often a side effect of a primary illness or condition rather than the primary health problem and is therefore ignored in treatment if not raised by the patient. As well as a biological problem, sexuality often involves psychological and social aspects that doctors aren't yet equipped to deal with.

Increasingly, clinical sexologists like Booysen are working with doctors to ensure sexual dysfunction associated with illness is addressed. Conditions in women such as endometriosis, vaginismus, vulvodynia and chronic pelvic pain can make penetrative sexual intercourse painful. Medications such as statins (used to treat high cholesterol), antidepressants, antipsychotics and even some hormonal birth control can all affect desire. But all kinds of sexual dysfunction can be treated. Pelvic physiotherapy can work wonders for women who experience pain during sex, or who have pelvic pain, endometriosis or vaginismus. And clinical sexologists may also be able to help in issues relating to desire and other types of sexual dysfunction.

ILLNESS AS CONTROL

But what about when illness is a patriarchal method of control? We saw in the chapter on hysteria how sex and sexual desire have both been put forward as causes and cures of illness. In *Complaints and Disorders: The sexual politics of sickness*, Barbara Ehrenreich and Deirdre English wrote of how being ill became almost fashionable for middle- and upper-class women in late nineteenth- and early twentieth-century America. 'Literature aimed at female readers lingered on the romantic pathos of illness and death; popular women's magazines featured such stories as "The Grave of My Friend" and "Song of Dying". Paleness and lassitude (along with filmy white gowns) came into vogue. It was acceptable, even fashionable, to retire to bed with "sick headaches", "nerves", and a host of other mysterious ailments.'[42] This was a convenient bonus for the coffers of medical professionals.

But female frailty also became a beauty ideal. 'The female consumptive did not lose her feminine identity, she embodied it: the bright eyes, translucent skin, and red lips were only an extreme of traditional female beauty,' write Ehrenreich and English.[43]

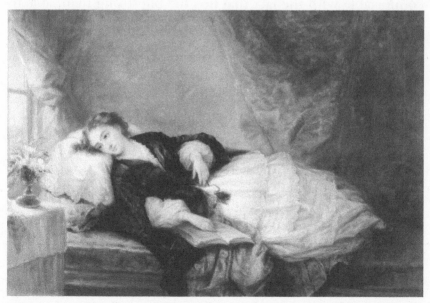

In the late nineteenth century, female frailty became a beauty ideal. This painting by Louis Lang is called *The Invalid* (1870).

And it was attractive in more than a physical sense. An idle wife was proof of a husband's wealth and success—a woman who could afford to be sick, after all, didn't need to make her own clothes, clean her house or look after children. The working-class women and women of colour who performed these chores were considered a breed apart: both sturdier and more robust but dirty and full of disease that could infect society.

A weak wife, one who needed to be cared for, added to her husband's sense of manliness. What's more, a weak and idle wife was unlikely to find another man. Where was the motivation, then, to find a cure or encourage recovery?

This phenomenon hasn't altogether disappeared. In fact, gynaecologist and pain specialist Dr Susan Evans tells me she sees it in her practice today in heterosexual couples where the wife has endometriosis or chronic pelvic pain. 'He's . . . comfortable with the fact that he's the big strong man, able to protect and care for and nurture her. And she's the vulnerable, weak woman who's very feminine and needs him in a big way. So where's the problem for him?' says Evans.

She's keen to point out that this behaviour is often subconscious and not vindictive. Society rewards men for their strength and ability to protect women. We're not talking about bad men, here; these are the messages received by good men—that their role is to, as Evans puts it, 'provide, protect and procreate'. 'That's really what they're about,' she says. 'They want to provide: home and hearth and food and things like that. And they want to protect [their wives] from risk and danger and bad things, and they want to be able to have sex and babies.'

The problem with these ideas of masculine protection, however, is they're so close to ownership. 'The ownership concept is very powerful for men,' Evans says. 'They like to think that she's "their" woman.' It's for this reason I've often had a problem with the messaging directed at men around domestic violence—much of it plays into the stereotypes that create the conditions for the violence to occur in the first place. At their worst, these go: 'You're the big strong man, you shouldn't be hitting this weak vulnerable woman, you should be protecting her!' I've always said to my partners: I don't want you to protect me, I want you to respect me.

This was put into sharp focus one evening when my boyfriend and I were dining at a trendy restaurant in Sydney. At the table next to us were four drunk men: two in their early 40s and two I guessed were their dads. One of the younger men, sitting closest to me, was extremely intoxicated, loud and obnoxious. He persistently tried to get my attention, at one point even throwing a bundle of fifty-dollar bills at me. I ignored him, which he obviously didn't like because he leant over and felt my breast.

Incensed, I yelled at him, 'How dare you touch me!'

He stuck his middle finger up at me and started calling me names as I kept yelling. The other younger man apologised and grabbed his friend, trying to calm him down.

I glanced at the older men, stunned at their silence, and said, 'That is sexual assault.' They looked away.

As I stood up to get the waiter's attention, two male staff arrived at the table to ask the men to leave the restaurant. When they rose, the older men apologised to my boyfriend, having never said a word to me—this enraged me more than having my breast groped!

My partner was angry about it, as angry as I was. But I was

grateful for how he handled it. He's a much calmer person than I am, and he stood back watching the situation, evaluating what needed to be done. He didn't need to do anything because the restaurant's staff acted so promptly and the men were gone within minutes, the situation diffused quickly and efficiently. I admired that he didn't get involved and turn it into an even bigger event.

But when I thanked him for his clear-headedness, he admitted to me that he felt guilty for not doing more— he felt 'unmanly' for not 'standing up' for me. He couldn't shake the idea that he should have punched my abuser. An Iranian-Australian, he said, 'If that had happened in Tehran, someone would have ended up dead.' And I said, 'Isn't that why you're glad you live in Australia?'

I reassured him that if he'd punched that man, I would have dumped him. I was happy with how the situation was handled. I certainly wasn't letting the imbecilic behaviour of a rich drunk white man ruin my evening—people like him have already ruined too much.

But when I recounted this story to friends, I was shocked by how many men said they would have punched the abuser. Men I admired, liked and respected felt it was their duty to meet undignified and abusive behaviour with violence—on behalf of 'their woman'. I still struggle to understand what a punch-up in an inner-city restaurant would have achieved. It wouldn't have made *me* feel better. But they can't help making the situation about *them*.

There's a strong cultural pressure on men to own, protect and defend their female partners at any cost—and many women buy into it. But I don't think that attitude can ever be synonymous with equality. In my relationship, we respect and protect each other. He watched me defend myself, stand up and call out the abuse; he didn't get involved when he wasn't needed because he respects my independence and admires my ability to look after myself. But a man needs maturity and confidence to be able to do that. (I've seen him run head-on into a brawl to break it up because he feared someone would be seriously hurt; I've seen him run to the scene of an accident to help victims. He's not afraid to get involved when *needed*.)

But it seems most men have little motivation to invest in ways to make women stronger and more independent. 'A vulnerable woman is someone he can feel good about supporting and protecting,' Evans tells me. 'It helps differentiate the thing that he's really comfortable with, which is the difference between men and women. He doesn't want to be the same, he doesn't want to be unisex, he wants to be "the man". And when you have a sick woman, it's like the vulnerability makes her even more feminine. I've seen lots of couples that come in where he seems very caring and nurturing. Her weakness is not actually a big deal, and he loves the fact that she needs him. She loves the fact that he looks after her.'

This isn't only about husbands who are controlling: it also upholds patriarchal structures and feeds into workplace issues. Sick women can't work or can't work full-time, and they have more sick days, which supports the idea that women are weaker than men, don't pull their weight at work and don't deserve equal pay.

As Kate Manne has shown in *Down Girl*, the control of women isn't always overt. Society as a whole plays a role in policing women, women included. The rewards for a woman who lives within the boundaries of her feminine role are rich—respect, appreciation, admiration, marriage and children. Putting the needs of others before her own is a defining characteristic of being a good woman. But the women with complex pain conditions are often not submissive; they sometimes put their own needs first. They don't accept the authority of the (usually) male doctor or the masculine tradition of medicine. They question his diagnosis, they 'doctor shop', they complain. As we'll find out in the next chapter, it's not just doctors who don't like these women, it's nurses and practice staff too. These women are threatening, not just medicine's claim to have complete knowledge of the human body, but society's long-held belief that women should suffer in silence and sacrifice their needs for the greater good.

This idea is further enforced by the two specific developments in a woman's illness that encourage action and place greater demands on doctors and politicians to do something: when the sick woman can't get pregnant and when she can't have sex because of pain. I'll give an example of each that shows how issues that affect men, when it comes to women's illnesses, are prioritised over those that affect only her.

First, let's consider how fertility often takes precedence as a symptom in endometriosis treatment, even when that is not the priority for the patient.[44]

I have endometriosis and adenomyosis, and I've had fertility problems, but even after undergoing IVF and trying to conceive for years, I still listed pain and fatigue ahead of fertility in order of treatment priority. In fact I stopped IVF treatment after three cycles because the impact on my quality of life was so intense, I couldn't stand to go through it again. If pain and fatigue were difficult to bear before IVF, they became almost unbearable during the cycles. Many other women say the same but some doctors continue to place fertility at the centre of endometriosis treatment without first consulting the patient. I have to say, this was not my experience—I have been lucky to have excellent doctors who have always put my needs and priorities at the centre of treatment. But Kate Young's research shows that the goal of medical treatment is often enabling a woman to have penis–vagina sex and fertility, without concern for the patient's treatment goals—these are more often to relieve symptoms that affect their quality of life, such as pain, fatigue, bladder and bowel problems, low mood and anxiety.[45] And it's even worse in some Asian countries, such as India, where endometriosis is usually only recognised and treated in cases of infertility. Of course fertility is important to many women, but it's prioritised over other symptoms because of its importance to men, especially in cultures where great weight is placed on being able to pass down the family name. And if an endometriosis patient doesn't have fertility issues—and most don't—her pain and other symptoms remain untreated.

But there's yet another factor in fertility that impacts unequal relationships between men and women. Most fertility research has focused solely on women, which has led to a common belief that women in Western countries are delaying childbirth because of their careers or other life goals. But a 2017 paper published in *Human Reproductive Update* found that in high-income countries, while as many men as women want to have children, women are delaying parenthood because of a lack of partner or lack of one willing to commit to parenthood. And this situation is driven by misinformation about male fertility.[46] Most men assume because they continue to produce sperm throughout their lives they can continue to produce offspring. High-profile older fathers such as Charlie Chaplin, who was 73 when his youngest son was born in 1962, and Robert De Niro, who was 68 when his youngest daughter was born in 2011, have helped give the impression that men are fertile forever—but this isn't true, and older dads may not be as common as once thought.

Several studies in recent years have shown conclusively that people with male reproductive organs have a biological clock.[47] While they continue producing sperm throughout their lives, its quality and quantity decreases with age, reducing its chances of achieving pregnancy and increasing the risk of miscarriage after the age of 40.[48] As a man ages, his sperm become corrupted by DNA damage, making his children more likely to have psychiatric and academic problems.[49] From age 45, his children are five times more likely to have an autism spectrum disorder and thirteen times more likely to be diagnosed with ADHD. A potential father or sperm donor's age negatively affects IVF success rates. In half the cases of infertility in the UK, people with male reproductive organs are the cause.[50] So it's beyond time male fertility became the focus of research and public education campaigns. And an end to hoary stereotypes about desperate women in their late 30s on the prowl for a husband and sperm donor. If men want to have healthy offspring, they should also be on the prowl at that age.

Now let's look at painful sex again. My example in this case comes from the reaction of some doctors when women complained that vaginal mesh implants made sex painful for them and it shows with depressing clarity how men are centred in women's pain.

The vaginal mesh scandal saw hundreds of thousands of women around the world surgically treated for prolapse of the pelvic organs—where the uterus, bladder or rectum move out of place because of a weakening of the pelvic floor muscles, ligaments or tissues, which is common after childbirth—with a product that had very little clinical evidence to support its effectiveness, often without women's full consent. One of the primary manufacturers of vaginal mesh products, Johnson & Johnson, has been accused of failing to conduct proper randomised controlled trials on the products and embarked on an aggressive marketing campaign to surgeons, who'd seen benefits in treating stress incontinence with similar products. The fact the devices were approved for pelvic organ prolapse with so little apparent evidence raises major questions about how seriously regulatory agencies around the world take women's health and wellbeing.

Vaginal mesh has caused life-altering pain and complications in hundreds of thousands of women globally. Class action lawsuits were brought by women against vaginal mesh manufacturers in Australia, the UK, US and Canada. 'More than 100,000 transvaginal mesh lawsuits have been filed in the US, with the manufacturer of the most commonly used meshes, Johnson & Johnson, facing the most lawsuits,' *The Guardian* reported in 2018.[51] Complications have included vaginal scarring, fistula formation, painful sex, and pelvic, back and leg pain; the mesh can also poke through the vaginal wall or cut through internal tissue. There are no official figures on how many women were treated with the product or official complication rates, but in the UK, NHS data suggests that one in fifteen women need to have their mesh surgically removed.[52]

How did the medical community react? Well, some gynae-cologists suggested these women should just try having anal sex instead. I wonder if they know of the research that suggests more than 70 per cent of women find anal sex painful.[53] Not that there's anything wrong with anal sex between consent-ing adults—indeed, Nina Booysen tells me that many of her female clients have found it an enjoyable alternative to vaginal sex. The offense is in the lack of regard to the issue of women being in pain, and the fact that even women who enjoy anal sex may not want this as their only long-term option. It assumes all the women involved are heterosexual. Also, for anyone with pelvic pain, anal intercourse can hurt just as much as vaginal intercourse. If female pleasure were top of mind, many non-penetrative options besides anal intercourse could be suggested. But instead of trying to resolve the pain and suffering of the women involved, these male doctors privileged the pleasure of the women's imagined male partners. Not to mention it wouldn't solve all the other pain and complications that vaginal mesh has caused. In addition to pain, many vaginal mesh victims suffer from what Shlomo Raz, a professor of urology and pelvic reconstruction at UCLA school of medicine, calls 'lupus-type' symptoms: runny nose, muscle pains, fogginess and lethargy.[54] How is anal sex to help with that?

This advice was exposed in an email exchange among French doctors working for Johnson & Johnson that emerged during the Australian class action against the company. One email went: 'I said to myself, there you go, for your next prolapse [patient], you talk to her about orgasms. OK! But also about fellatio, sodomy, the clitoris with or without G-spot etc. I am sure of one thing: that I would very quickly be treated like some kind of sex maniac (which, perhaps, I am) or a pervert, or an unhealthily curious person.'[55] Note the mention of fellatio but not cunnilingus. Whose pleasure is this doctor primarily concerned with?

The fact a gynaecologist would consider it inappropriate to discuss sex with a patient, when so many gynaecological problems can affect the sex lives of people with female sex organs, is a sign of the enormous size of our society's problem with talking about sex. This has to change, and doctors— who play a leading role in society—should be trained to speak about this aspect of our innate humanity openly and without embarrassment. Kate Young's research finds that many doctors still struggle with it, believing it's someone else's job to fix.

Anyone may be embarrassed to report painful sex to a doctor, not knowing it's a symptom of many other conditions, and not considering sexual health as part of overall health. Investing in ourselves as sexual beings—even if it means choosing not to have sex—can affect our health: physical, mental and biological. A healthy sex life—whatever that means for you—is consistently shown to be an important factor in quality-of-life measures, and to understand and be confident in our sexuality is part of being a healthy, vibrant human.

CHAPTER 5

It's the culture, stupid: understanding modern medical practice

Family violence, particularly in a small-town context. And all the things that go with that, so not just the physical violence, the emotional abuse, the financial abuse, finding ways to help people escape that—women escape that— within the constraints of a small town is to me, the hardest thing I do . . . There's the physical trauma stuff but the bigger part I see is the psychological trauma, the fall out of years and years of post-traumatic stress disorder even once women have left a violent home. The women who've grown up as kids in a violent home struggling with their own sense of self because the only way they've ever viewed their sense of self-worth is through the eyes of their abuser—that sort of stuff I find really really challenging and it's very very easy for the mental health services in particular to label them as a borderline personality disorder, which is a women's diagnosis. Borderline is a women's diagnosis and once it's made, mental health services say, 'They're just borderline, there's nothing we can do. They need DBT.'

There is one person who provides [dialectical behaviour therapy] in [the region], privately. Community mental health doesn't provide it at all. In-patient mental health doesn't provide it at all. So once they make that diagnosis, these are women, usually, who are chronically suicidal, chronically self-harming, really high risk, and mental health just say, 'Oh they're borderliners, they're manipulative, they're this, they're that.'

It's not a helpful diagnosis. It is victim blaming . . . it puts it completely back on them: 'They're just being manipulative.' It's the modern form of hysteria. It's just *their* problem. We don't need to take responsibility as a society, we don't need to do anything about it, we don't need to provide services to manage it. Stuff 'em, they're just manipulative, they're just hysterical, they're just just just.

This is how Anita Saldanha, a GP working in an Australian small town a hundred kilometres from the nearest referral hospital, responds when I ask her about the hardest part of her job. We're sitting at her dining-room table looking out over rolling hills, brown from a lack of rain but still beautiful. I ask her if she's read Jane Ussher's book, *The Madness of Women*, in which she comes to similar conclusions about borderline personality disorder, also describing it as a modern form of hysteria, and points to a study that found 86 per cent of women with a borderline personality disorder diagnosis had been sexually abused.[1] She hasn't but she's not surprised at the statistic—it marries with what she sees in her practice. Before I began work on this book, I didn't know anything about borderline personality disorder; I wasn't focused on mental health, I was focused on pain. But doctor after doctor raised it with me.

Another GP, Clare Fairweather, who works in an Australian capital city, calls borderline personality disorder a 'pejorative diagnosis' and tells me, 'It's such a dangerous label to apply to young women.' She says some doctors see it as a get-out-of-gaol-free card because once they view the diagnosis on the patient's history, all the woman's symptoms can be seen 'through the prism of their naughty personality'. 'A young woman presenting with borderline personality disorder in the emergency department will not be treated nicely, will not be taken seriously, and she's in danger because of that.' Fairweather says a prevalent attitude in medicine goes: 'They're just seeking, they're just hysterical, they're just borderline, get them out of my emergency room.' A male physician who has worked in emergency departments throughout urban and rural New South Wales and Queensland categorically supports this assessment.

Fairweather thinks young women and girls are being diagnosed with borderline personality disorder too early, when their personalities are still emerging, and that boys and men the same age with similar symptoms are usually given a more medically respected diagnosis: often treatment-resistant depression, a condition taken more seriously and one with better treatment options. Two male GPs working in rural Australia tell me it is also their impression that some young women are diagnosed with borderline personality disorder at too young an age.

Women make up more than 75 per cent of borderline personality disorder diagnoses, and there isn't much clinical guidance for effective treatment. Fairweather points out borderline personality disorder is gendered not only in who gets diagnosed but also in how it's diagnosed: 'The other gendered aspect of borderline personality disorder is that one of the formulations for the genesis of the borderline personality is that it occurs because of disordered attachment in infancy. It's often seen through a lens of trauma and abuse so therefore sexual abuse, or more commonly, a hostile mother.' The echoes of hysteria are loud, as loud as medicine's role as the moral guardian of current social mores: a mother who doesn't conform to the idealised feminine role of devoted, giving parent and servant is in modern times blamed for the mental distress of her children.

But we can't forget that the suffering of people with borderline personality disorder is very real. While Rachael Tait, a British GP working in Norfolk, says that services and support for people with borderline personality disorder are hard to come by in the NHS, she tells me about a patient who found the diagnosis a positive experience, 'For her, it was an explanation for why she was the way that she was,' Tait says. She agrees that it's a gendered diagnosis but thinks that in older women, it's probably underdiagnosed.

Since the meaning of hysteria has always reflected social conditions, we shouldn't be surprised to see it among us today as symptoms of sexual trauma or violence. What surprises me from my research and interviews isn't the consensus that emerged of borderline personality disorder as the modern form of hysteria, but how many conditions were raised and put forward by doctors and academics to fit this label.

Whenever treatment options are limited because of a lack of medical understanding of how a condition works, hysteria narratives start to emerge. Women are blamed for their own illnesses—sometimes because of their supposed mental instability, sometimes because of choices such as delaying childbirth. Borderline personality disorder, endometriosis, chronic pelvic pain, fibromyalgia, chronic fatigue syndrome have all been put forward by the medical profession as conditions with a high prevalence of hysterical, difficult or crazy patients. That the majority of them are women isn't the only thing these conditions have in common—the other is that medical knowledge is severely limited, with no cure and no proven or effective long-term treatment available.

How did we get here?

IS HEALTHCARE SEXIST?

Of course healthcare is sexist—society is sexist. It would be a miracle if one of Western civilisation's most exclusive institutions—medicine—were not. But we're not here to condemn medicine or to bash doctors. Western healthcare systems don't ignore women or minimise their suffering because doctors are sexist. No doubt some are—and medicine undoubtedly has a problem weeding these doctors out, even those who do harm to their patients[2]—but most doctors want to help their patients. It would be easy to improve women's health if the problems were all caused by a few sexist pigs—but as with all discrimination, sexism in medicine is structural. Institutions, especially those as old and exclusive as medicine, are inherently conservative because they exist to support the status quo. Understanding how sexism works in medicine is important because it has such profound effects on our health. Along with religion and politics, medicine has historically played an integral role in policing and controlling women. As an institution, it still does today.

By looking at how medicine is practised, I hope we can better understand how to dismantle the structures that deprioritise women's health.

IS WOMEN'S HEALTH REALLY ALL THAT BAD?

Women have always lived longer than men on average, across cultures. It was once assumed this was due to the fact men are risk-takers and die younger from accidents, workplace injuries and war. But researchers have found that this doesn't fully account for the disparity in life expectancy. The shocking truth is, nobody knows why women live longer than men.

Some scientists believe the female immune system could play a role. We know it's stronger and more flexible than the male one, protecting life from its earliest stages, with female premature babies showing consistently stronger survival rates than male ones.[3] So much for the weaker sex, right? But this flexibility means there's more scope for things to go wrong, and women pay for this with conditions of the immune system. 'Men die quicker, women are sicker,' goes an old adage among medical professionals.

Women account for three-quarters of people with auto-immune conditions, and for a huge proportion of the global burden of pain. They're more likely to suffer from persistent pain than men—a 2008 multi-country study found the prevalence for chronic pain was 45 per cent of women and 31 per cent of men.[4] In all chronic pain conditions, there's a substantial prevalence of women. That's not to say men don't experience chronic pain, but while its distribution evens out in old age, women experience it more during their reproductive years, and so it has a huge impact on their opportunities and quality of life.

As Maya Dusenbery reports in *Doing Harm*, 'When it comes to "active" life expectancy—the number of years living free from significant limitations that prevent you from doing everyday tasks—men have overtaken women over the past three decades. Women still live longer, but men live *better* longer.'[5]

The conditions that affect a higher proportion of women than men are also among the most under-researched, creating a gap in medical understanding that affects how women are treated and perceived by health professionals. This alone would probably mean that women go to the doctor more frequently than men. But women not only have to see doctors when they're sick, they're also often obliged to go for other reasons, as I've already mentioned.

Some of these interactions involve health risks, and medical intervention might be necessary. But there's no good evidence, for example, to support continued doctor visits over many years of taking the birth control pill. In 2017 when New Zealand made the pill available over-the-counter at pharmacies after an initial GP assessment, the move was supported by the Royal Australian and New Zealand College of Obstetricians and Gynaecologists. The same move was proposed during an Australian state election in 2018 and was supported by women's reproductive health NGOs such as Plan International and Marie Stopes. But the Australian Medical Association—the peak body for doctors—opposed the proposal because it 'would be a missed opportunity for preventative health screening and checks that go along with going to a doctor for a repeat script'.[6] Try to imagine a major medical organisation forcing men to go to the doctor for a condom prescription just as a method of checking up on them.

One experienced male physician tells me to investigate why doctors must be involved in dispensing the morning-after pill—which, he says 'is safer than Panadol'. There's simply no case for requiring a medical prescription for the morning-after pill, he says, other than an attempt to restrict access. Other hormonal contraceptives require medical skills for insertion, like IUDs and Implanon, but after insertion, you're on your own for months or years at a time, so why not with the pill? The oral contraceptive pill and the morning-after pill could easily be dispensed by licensed pharmacists with some control measures put in place.

He also urges me to investigate why abortion isn't routinely performed in Australian public hospitals. 'If it's a legal right, it should be performed in the public system,' he says. While abortions should obviously be performed by doctors—even medical abortions (those caused by taking a tablet) require medical monitoring because of the health risks involved—they should be performed by *more* doctors. In other words, there's an imbalance between forcing women to see doctors when it's unnecessary for their health and forcing doctors to see women when it is necessary for their health.

The near-constant interactions that women must have with health professionals over the course of their lives means the relationship between a woman and her doctor is important. But these interactions take place in a sexist society, which influences this relationship.

Gynaecologist and pain physician Dr Susan Evans is adamant that healthcare is sexist—but not because doctors hate women. Rather, she says, it's an accumulation of lots of 'little things'. 'It's everything from our cultural backgrounds, which haven't been pro-women; it's the fact that women's pain is pain you can't see; the fact that our society in general doesn't listen to women; it's the fact that pain symptoms are described [by women] in ways that men don't appreciate; it's the non-prioritising of issues of importance to women, and that covers the undervaluing of gynaecology compared to other specialities,' she says. 'So it's in the undervaluing of the skills [involved in treating women], it's the undervaluing of listening, it's the lack of provision of services . . .; it's the lack of women in decision-making roles . . .; it's the sexual connotations that women are not supposed to talk about things "down there"; it's the economic ability of women to pay for things, which is diminished . . . The add up is not that anybody is particularly mean and nasty, it's just that every step of the way, the women's stuff is deprioritised.'

HYSTERIA IN MODERN MEDICINE

I documented the history of hysteria in Chapter 3 in order to highlight the foundations of medical knowledge when it comes to women's health. Institutional knowledge isn't re-invented with every generation; new research builds on what's already known or understood. Of course, mistakes and mis-understandings get corrected—this happens continually in medical science—but because knowledge of female biology remains so far behind that of male biology, hysteria is an old habit that dies hard.

For the purposes of understanding medical practice today, this lack of knowledge on female biology is troublesome because of the power of doctors, who tend to be viewed by society as knowing the truth about the human body.[7] Public health researcher, Dr Kate Young has uncovered how doctors fill knowledge gaps with hysteria narratives. This is particularly prevalent when women keep returning to the doctor, stubbornly refusing to be saved. 'The historical hysteria discourse was most often endorsed when discussing "difficult" women, referring to those for whom treatment was not helpful or who held a perception of their disease alternative to their clinician,' Young has written. 'Rather than acknowledge the limitations of medical knowledge, medicine expected women to take control (with their minds) of their disease (in their body) by accepting their illness, making "lifestyle" changes, and conforming to their gendered social roles of wife and mother. Moralising discourses surround those who rebel; they are represented as irrational and irresponsible, the safety net for medicine when it cannot fulfil its claim to control the body.'[8] A male GP once earnestly said to me, 'I've never had a fibromyalgia patient who wasn't batshit crazy.'

In her work, Young has shown how endometriosis patients are often viewed by their treating doctors as 'reproductive bodies with hysterical tendencies'.[9] In this case, patients aren't being diagnosed with a psychological illness and thrown in the medical wastebasket; they are diagnosed with a painful physical disease but treated as though they brought it on themselves, or that they refuse to get better because they like being sick. It's to Young that the gynaecologist I quoted in the introduction said: 'Do mad people get endo or does endo make you mad? It's probably a bit of both.' Another said, 'there's a lot of psychology, just as much as there is pathology [in gynaecology]'.[10]

Other research has shown that in gynaecological literature, endometriosis patients were presented as having a 'disordered personality and behaviour' as well as 'disordered female biology'.[11] Nobody suggests that endometriosis isn't a real disease, or is somehow imagined, but there is a general feeling in medicine that women's reaction to having endometriosis is somehow hysterical, especially when symptoms prevail after treatment has been offered, which is common.

But medical practice itself often induces the distress that leads to the emotional behaviour doctors despair over. The tendency to prioritise fertility in treatment, as discussed in the previous chapter, often increases anxiety among young women, adding to the idea that endometriosis patients and women in general 'catastrophise', and are difficult patients. Clare Fairweather sees this in her practice regularly. 'When [fertility] is prioritised, when there's a lot of chat about that, it terrifies them. OK, they don't want a baby now, but they're all very worried that they're not going to be able to ever have a baby, which is just not true.' While official figures claim that about a third of endo patients are infertile, recent research by Young puts the figure at a much lower rate of 10 to 13 per cent.[12] 'Don't escalate their anxieties and fears by something that might never happen,' Fairweather warns. 'It's pointless dwelling on that if that's not what they wish to have addressed at this moment.'

Sylvia Freedman, co-founder of the Australian advocacy group EndoActive, has written about how she reacted when her gynaecologist told her that she had to have a baby young or miss out altogether.[13]

I was falling behind at uni and missing work because of pain. I needed relief from my symptoms but my doctor was focused on my fertility. I was young, ill-informed and desperate to be 'cured' . . . and desperation will do crazy things to a person.

Like most girls, I had spent my entire sexually active life trying not to get pregnant. Now all of a sudden I'm thinking I may never have kids but if I want them at all I should get cracking.

I spent months plotting ways of becoming pregnant. I was broke, in pain, still living at home. And single. And all I could think was: 'So who's going to be my baby daddy?'

There was no time to waste on Tinder but nothing a gay best friend and a turkey baster couldn't fix. I quickly got on the phone to make sure I had sperm if I needed it. I even got my family on board: 'If you want grandkids, now's the time. Got any friends with gay sons? Call them. Now. We may need their spawn.'

In hindsight, I am disturbed by the lengths I went to. I was tortured. How can you look after a baby when you're too sick to look after yourself?

In her advocacy and research work, Freedman has spoken to thousands of women with endo who've reported being told by their doctor that pregnancy is a cure, or that they must have children young if they want to at all; their doctor then prioritised treating fertility before pain and other symptoms. One girl commented on EndoActive's Facebook page: 'My doctor told me having a baby would help my pain. I'm only eleven.' And another: 'My GP told me to go to the pub and have a one night stand and try to get pregnant before I missed the boat.'

Pain relief is often the priority for women with endo and chronic pelvic pain. The pain can be scary, especially for young women—not being able to get out of bed to go to school, university or work is difficult. Waiting years for a diagnosis is hard. Not being believed, or having your pain minimised, is challenging. Trying treatment after treatment that doesn't work is physically and mentally draining. As Saldanha says to me: 'Chronic pain makes you crazy. It gets into your head.' Fairweather points out: 'Teenagers . . . don't have much life experience at this point, the pain is quite a catastrophic thing for them, and they're frightened.'

When I was first diagnosed with endometriosis in 2001, I was relieved to have an answer after years of thinking I was just weak. Trying to understand more about it, I jumped online to look for support groups. What I found horrified me. Comment after comment from women who'd given up work, who hadn't been able to have sex for years, divorces, relationship breakdowns, unaffordable treatments, poverty, financial ruin, whole lives of singledom—because of pain! Each story was more tragic than the last. But I'd just had surgery and was feeling better. My doctor promised me I'd feel better for years. I didn't want to become one of those 'whingeing women'. I didn't want to be sick. I didn't want to be a drag.

I logged off and didn't join another endo group until Endo-Active came along.

What I didn't understand then but do now is that those women weren't complaining because they were born miserable: they were complaining because they have a disease that has few effective treatment options and wide ignorance among medical practitioners of best practice options; even the caring doctors aren't always up to speed with the latest pain treatments.

Rich women can doctor shop. I'm not rich but I am fairly privileged and I was able to do my research to find an endo specialist who'd spent his career trying to help women with the disease. But many other women—and endo doesn't discriminate along race or class lines—can be stuck with a doctor who doesn't believe them. Women of colour are often written off as drug seekers. Poor women are suspected of wanting to get out of work. Rich women are perfectionists or merely anxious. Overweight women just need to lose weight. People who are gender transitioning have hormonal issues.

So, um, yes: endometriosis patients, and other people with chronic pain conditions—men who suffer from diseases with a knowledge gap frequently fare poorly too—are sometimes difficult. Often they know it. Fairweather says, 'They start to perceive themselves as being unable to cope and as being inherently broken and having really crappy coping mechanisms.' Deep in the collective knowledge of women is that doctors have the power to label them as 'crazy' or to dismiss them entirely, notions that scare many sufferers out of seeking treatment. A 2014 study published in *Circulation* journal found that women delayed seeking treatment when they suspected they were having a heart attack, partly because they were worried about being seen as a hypochondriac if they were wrong.[14]

For women of colour or other minority status, this fear can feel more life-threatening than the illness itself. There's a long history of Aboriginal women having their children removed from them when they present for medical care; a mental health diagnosis could result in the separation of their families. Young tells me: 'In my study, I spoke to women from very diverse backgrounds and almost all of them spoke about how they often felt scared or anxious about the power that their doctor had over them in terms of when they were knocked out and in surgery, or if their doctor decided they didn't believe what they were saying, they denied them access to healthcare, or a few of them spoke about their ability to label them as crazy as well.'

We should be aware that fear and anxiety arising from interactions with doctors could be exacerbating patients' pain. As Saldanha notes: 'We know that there's a relationship between pain and mood, we know that when mood is worse that pain will be worse, we know that when pain is worse, mood will be worse. They're interrelated issues—you can't treat one without treating the other.'

But there's a wider social problem here too, as Kate Manne explains in *Down Girl*: '[A woman] will tend to be in trouble when she does not give enough, or to the right people, in the right way, or in the right spirit. And, if she errs on this score, or asks for something of the same support or attention on her own behalf, there is a risk of misogynist resentment, punishment, and indignation.'[15] These women *are* asking for care, support, treatment and they're asking to be believed.

Evans helps explain why chronic pain patients so often get the 'difficult' label: 'A lot of the women who have had pain for a long time, they really are quite challenging . . . They cry a lot. It doesn't actually worry me but it's quite off-putting for some people. And also they have so many symptoms that you think you've done well with one, and yet then there's the next one and the next one and next one.' She also points out that often it isn't the doctors themselves labelling these patients as difficult but nursing and practice administrative staff. 'Some of them ring up a lot, needy, teary, desperate—you don't blame them, they are! But the staff don't like them, the nurses don't like them. The hospitals don't like them because they hang around longer in hospital beds. No one particularly wants them and that is so sad.'

Evans believes that part of the problem is the language women use to describe their pain. A 2009 study published in the *Pain* journal found that women tend to use more words and more graphic language, and focus on the sensory aspects of pain; men tend to use fewer words and less descriptive language, and focus on events and emotions.[16] The effect is that women can be seen as dramatic and emotional when describing their pain, especially in a male-dominated environment such as medicine. Even female doctors, after training and working in the heavily masculinised medical culture, can view this language as confronting and histrionic.

Women in pain aren't the only difficult patients. Those with borderline personality disorder—of all genders—often have a history of trauma and tough life circumstances, have faced delays with diagnosis, and have faced doctor after doctor shrugging their shoulders and not knowing what to do with them. Borderline personality disorder and pain patients can be very difficult to deal with, but this is partly because they lack effective treatments for their conditions.

Saldanha recalls a time when this happened to her: 'I can remember being a junior doctor in emergency and being so pleased when I finally lost my temper at the borderline patient who'd presented for the fourth time, four shifts running and she refused to see me. She said, "I won't see that black bitch anymore" . . . I can remember being so relieved that someone else had to deal with her. And that's awful. That's not me at all. But I was just so tired and so under pressure and felt so bottom rung that I was relieved that that poor girl wouldn't see me. I mean, she was seventeen and she wanted to kill herself. For fuck's sake, what was I thinking?'

Doctors often use the term 'heartsink patients' to describe people like this teenage girl and other patients with complex problems. Rachael Tait says it's often people of lower socio-economic background, with complex health problems and lifestyle issues who get put into the heartsink category. She says, 'When you're looking at patients who are already really entrenched with these problems, to be honest, I think a lot of people almost write them off and see them as hopeless cases.' They're the ones with depression, fibromyalgia and chronic fatigue syndrome, who don't go away, who never get better. They *are* hard to treat because not enough research has been done on their conditions. Many doctors don't like them. Other doctors believe diagnoses such as fibromyalgia and chronic fatigue syndrome are harmful labels because there's no good treatment and it stigmatises the patient. Three different doctors told me fibromyalgia was an unhelpful label—not because they didn't believe the patient was ill, quite the opposite, because they believed other medical practitioners wouldn't take the patient seriously with that diagnosis or else would just give them opiates which could make their problems worse. Young's research suggests that doctors don't label patients as hysterical or difficult with the intention of subordinating them—it's just that their medical education taught them they knew all about the human body and that it's their job to fix people. This is why Young and her colleagues have argued that it's the culture of medicine we need to address, not individual clinicians.

Young explains the doctor's dilemma to me: 'Doctors feel a lot of pressure to provide their patients with answers no matter what . . . normally something very tangible like a drug or a surgery. And when they don't have an answer, it seems to be in the case of endometriosis, that they draw upon these really repressive medical discourses and they look for a fault within the women themselves, and they say, "well this isn't my fault, this is your fault, it's clearly something you're doing, a choice in your life, you're not trying hard enough, you're not exercising enough, you took too long to have a baby", or—a classic—"the symptoms must be in your head. I've done everything that the text books and papers have told me to do and now I can't do it anymore."'

MEDICAL EDUCATION

Not enough is done in Western medical education to prepare doctors to deal with patients whose symptoms can't be resolved or relieved with current medical care. '[We're taught] either you can fix people or you can palliate people but there's this whole section of the community who live in the grey area in between,' Saldanha told me.

Saldanha, Fairweather, Evans and two other country doctors I've chosen not to name all told me that nothing in their medical education equipped them to adequately treat patients with chronic pain conditions and psychological disorders such as borderline personality disorder. 'No health professional finishes their training with all the skills required to care for [chronic pelvic pain patients],' Evans says.

Medical students aren't routinely taught about the male-centred bias of medical knowledge, or encouraged to analyse how stereotypes of women and minority groups may influence their impression of patients. There are few lessons, if any, on medical uncertainty or training on how to manage difficult patients. It's encouraging to see some postgraduate training being offered to doctors around Australia on dealing with 'heartsink' patients and managing chronic pain. While there's some education on chronic diseases, curricula focus mainly on asthma, diabetes and cardiovascular disease, and there's nothing to tell students that almost all knowledge of these diseases comes from studies conducted by men, on men, even though it's now widely understood that biology plays a major role in influencing how a disease presents itself and how drugs work.

As I've mentioned already, cardiovascular disease is now well understood to present differently in women and men, but students aren't necessarily being told to look out for this. The result is that women are frequently sent home with anxiety diagnoses, or no diagnosis at all, while suffering heart attacks.

An American study conducted by the psychologist Gabrielle Chiaramonte illustrates how sexist assumptions show up in the diagnosis of heart disease. The study of more than 200 doctors involved male and female patients with the same symptoms, but adding a stressful life event dramatically altered how the patient was diagnosed. While diagnoses were fairly consistent before the stressful life event was mentioned, after its mention only 15 per cent of medical students or residents diagnosed heart disease in the woman compared to 56 per cent for the man, and only 30 per cent referred the woman to a cardiologist compared to 62 per cent for the man. Only 13 per cent suggested cardiac medication for the woman, versus 47 per cent for the man. Remember, these patients presented with exactly the same symptoms—including the stressful life event. Once that was mentioned, diagnoses shifted from an organic cause (a disease) to a psychogenic one in women but not men. Women were assumed to be suffering from nothing but anxiety, while for the men the stressful event supported the diagnosis of heart disease since stress is a risk factor. The doctor's gender didn't influence results.[17]

One American cardiologist said it clearly in an interview: 'In training, we were taught to be on the lookout for hysterical females who come to the emergency room.'[18]

Addressing the imbalance of knowledge on female biology is urgent, and telling medical students about this knowledge bias is essential if women are to be treated better. Some major medical schools, such as Harvard, have introduced a social medicine course in order to address the social determinants of health and equip young doctors to think critically about their role in patients' lives, including how a patient's life circumstances may be influencing their illness and symptoms or the doctor's view of those symptoms. But Kate Young says, while this course is great, it still fails to address the male bias of medical knowledge.

It's a start, at least, and there's a sense among academics that the success of the Harvard course will see it spread to other medical schools around the world. But even at Harvard, the course was at first resisted by students, who didn't understand how learning about this stuff, not to mention medical uncertainty, would help them become better doctors. Most medical schools still only talk about medical uncertainty briefly. 'I find that fascinating,' Young says, 'because we're only human, of course we're not going to understand how every single aspect of the body works. I think they realise, on the first day on the job, that they don't have all the answers, and medicine isn't black and white but it's all grey. But it's still hard, because no one's ever really said to them, "There are going to be lots of patients coming to you for help and you're not going to know how to help them, and it's not their fault, just because you don't know." I think they find that very confronting.'

MEDICAL CULTURE

The culture within medicine leaves little room for uncertainty: 'the price of success is conformity', says Young. As a profession it has a well-known culture of discrimination, bullying and harassment. A third of medical trainees experience sexual harassment internationally.[19] In the US, doctors commit suicide at rates higher than any other profession,[20] with similar results found in other Western nations.[21] In Australia, female doctors, as well as male and female nurses and midwives, commit suicide at much higher rates than the rest of the workforce.[22] In 2015, an Australian vascular surgeon, Dr Gabrielle

McMullin, sparked headlines by saying that sexism was so rife in surgical training that women would be better off accepting sexual advances by senior staff than reporting them. Referring to a female surgeon, Dr Caroline Tan, who had been vilified and unable to get a job in Australia after making a successful sexual harassment claim, McMullin said in an interview with the ABC: 'Her career was ruined by this one guy asking for sex on this night. And, realistically, she would have been much better to have given him a blow job on that night.'[23] The hierarchical nature of medicine, and the way career development depends on references and recommendations from senior staff, means that harassment and abuse are rarely reported. Sexual harassment and the routine humiliation of junior doctors is normalised within the culture.[24]

'If you speak up and say my supervisor sexually assaulted me, your name's going to be mud,' Saldanha tells me. 'Getting a training place is going to be impossible.' This received knowledge perpetuates a cycle of non-reporting. In 2015, the Royal Australasian College of Surgeons commissioned an investigation into workplace culture following the Caroline Tan case, and it revealed entrenched bullying and harassment in surgery and other medical disciplines. The college introduced a new policy against discrimination, bullying and harassment that other Australian colleges also adopted. But Louise Stone, a GP and clinical associate professor at the Australian National University Medical School, has found that the new policies haven't done much to encourage women to report sexual abuse. In a context where wider society, including the justice system, doesn't take sexual harassment and assault claims seriously, and where junior doctors witness daily the contradiction between policies and accepted behaviour, there's little incentive to come forward, she claimed in an article for *MJA InSight*.[25]

And it's not just about sexual harassment. Men—particularly non-white, LGBTI+ or immigrant men—suffer too if they don't accept the bullying or comply with the oppressive culture. 'I can't help thinking that the hidden shame of medicine may yet turn out to be the doctor–doctor relationship, that powerful force which ultimately influences how doctors treat their patients,' Dr Ranjana Srivastava, an oncologist, wrote in *The Guardian*. 'Do doctors argue, fuss and fight? Do they have trouble working with each other in genuine collaboration? Absolutely. The medical profession as a whole abounds with fragile egos and deep vulnerabilities.' She outlines the feudal wars present in the system: 'researchers hate clinicians as people who feed off their intellect. Clinicians scoff at lab doctors who don't inhabit the real world. And clinician-researchers, derided for being too much of one or the other, are never sure where they belong. General practitioners are sick of the condescension from specialists. Specialists tussle among themselves and with entrenched hierarchies.'[26]

One effect is increasing levels of anxiety, depression and suicide among doctors. But I've heard doctors defend the brutal culture by saying medical practitioners need to have high resilience. That's interesting—why is it that female and minority doctors seem to be required to have higher resilience than the privileged white straight male doctors who are the primary enforcers and beneficiaries of that culture? Few of those men are discriminated against, bullied or harassed. In 2017, after four junior doctors took their own lives within the space of six months in Australia, as an editor at *The Guardian*

Australia I commissioned some reporting to reflect on medicine's training culture. One writer I commissioned, Georgina Dent, wrote about the brutal toll medical training takes:

> Training positions are scarce and the stakes are high. There are interviews, exams, research and courses to undertake on top of working 100-plus hours a week in busy public hospitals where, almost invariably, there are more patients than doctors can see.
>
> By the time a young doctor has decided on a particular speciality to train in, the work required to give them even a whiff of hope of securing a training position in that field necessarily limits their other options.
>
> If all of your work placements, research, study, contacts and exams are for one speciality and you miss out, you will need to start from scratch to establish credibility and experience in another.
>
> It is daunting for anyone who has spent years dedicating themselves to their career, to face the reality of falling short. And yet it happens.
>
> For almost every speciality, there is only one chance a year to qualify. Have a bad interview and it's another whole year to wait. Fail to pass the primary exam required to get an interview? Another whole year. And another $3,000 or $4,000 for the privilege.[27]

We also asked doctors to share with us, anonymously if they wished, their mental health struggles. The responses were harrowing: people dreaming about dead babies; struggling with alcohol and other addictions; self-medicating because reporting a mental health issue would be career ending; and suffering from depression, anxiety, bullying, sexual harassment, racism, snobbery, humiliation. Countless careers ruined after reporting harassment or bullying, jobs lost after seeking support for mental health issues. Doctors who are under so much pressure they end up hating their patients.

But apparently it's all par for the course in medical training—anybody who can't cope doesn't deserve to be there. This was certainly the message received from the medical culture by the vast majority of the hundred-odd people who responded to our call-out.

A 2013 survey of thousands of Australian doctors confirmed what we were reading. It found that one in five medical students and one in ten doctors had suicidal thoughts in the past year. It revealed doctors experience high psychological distress at much greater rates than the general population, high rates of alcohol abuse and an entrenched stigma against mental health issues.[28]

As Srivastava has pointed out, this culture has an effect on patient care. But it also means change arrives at a glacial pace and that ancient thinking is passed down. Student doctors are learning their profession in a fiercely competitive environment where questioning is punished and conformity rewarded. Is it any wonder that doctors blame patients when they don't have answers?

And yet, things are changing. A greater number of women in medical practice and research has helped. The women's health movement that swept through the West in the 1970s and 80s drew attention to the widespread lack of knowledge of female biology and managed to change US laws to include women in clinical trials that changed medical science around the world. Research showed the importance of a good bedside manner and listening to patients, and there are now many more doctors practising in a patient-centred way. But those doctors, and the skills required to achieve this kind of care, are still vastly undervalued.

WOMEN'S SKILLS AND WOMEN'S HEALTH PROCEDURES UNDERVALUED

While women now make up half of medical students in Australia, the US and the UK, the medical hierarchy has barely changed. With a majority of female medical students for two decades, parity in specialisation should have been reached by 2008.[29] However, only 34 per cent of Australian specialists are female, and women make up 10 per cent of surgeons.[30] In Australia, female GPs are paid on average 25 per cent less than their male colleagues.[31] In 2018, female GPs earnt 33 per cent less than male GPs in the UK.[32] In the US, data from 2018 showed that female doctors earn an average of 27.7 per cent less than their male peers.[33] These figures are remarkably similar, extraordinary considering the different healthcare systems in place in these countries. And in all three countries, the gap has actually widened in recent years, despite the fact that female doctors perform equally as well as their male peers on measures of medical knowledge, communication skills, professionalism, technical skills, practice-based learning and clinical judgement.[34]

In fact, research shows that patients are more likely to survive a heart attack if treated by a female doctor. When those patients are women, they're three times more likely to survive if their doctor is female than if he is male,[35] while another study showed female doctors have more empathy than male doctors and that probably makes them better doctors.[36] In 2016 Harvard researchers found that when elderly patients were treated by female doctors in hospital, they were less likely to die or to return to hospital after discharge.[37] This research shows not only do female doctors save lives, but they save healthcare systems money. So why are they paid less?

A number of factors are at play. Women earn less even when hours of work are accounted for, so it's not just about them working part-time or fewer hours. The fields of medicine that women have usually been attracted to are paid the least and are the most undervalued; women have gravitated towards general practice (or family medicine), pathology, paediatrics, and obstetrics and gynaecology—supporting the idea that anything to do with women and children is inferior. Surgeons tend to earn the highest salaries of all medical professionals, and even though gynaecologists are surgeons, their urology counterparts tend to earn much higher pay cheques. Women are underrepresented in leadership roles at hospitals and medical schools—again, this is common across Australia, the US and UK. Some of the higher paid specialities, such as surgery, have been almost entirely reserved for men through a highly masculinised culture that can be off-putting to women and prohibits a balance between work and caring responsibilities in training.[38] After an Australian junior doctor, Chloe Abbott, killed herself in 2017, her sister Micaela told News.com.au, 'Very early on, when Chloe was at university, they were told if you want to be a female doctor and you want to still have children, the only path you should go down is GP training.'

Since women make up just over half of GPs in Australia, let's look at this speciality for an example of how bias against women's health and female medical professionals is deeply entrenched.

In 2018, an inner-Melbourne medical practice kicked off a media storm when it put up a sign announcing female GPs would be charging more than male GPs because women's health issues take longer to deal with than men's, and women tend to self-select female doctors. A patient seeing a female GP at the clinic would now pay $44.95, after Medicare's fee, and a patient seeing a male GP would be $37.95 out of pocket for a standard consultation. Social media went into overdrive. General sentiment went: Women already pay more for their health with costs of menstruation and contraception; they earn less, have more chronic health issues and need to see the doctor more. How is it fair for them to be charged more?

Obviously it isn't fair but it serves to highlight other unfairnesses in the system, such as, although female GPs have better patient outcomes because they spend more time on preventative health than their male counterparts, they earn significantly less than them. Australian GPs are paid by Medicare per consultation, and what Medicare values is highly skewed towards the skills men tend to have—such as skin excisions—and women's health procedures, and the provision of preventative and psychosocial care, which women tend to be good at, are vastly undervalued.[39]

Let's look at some examples of women's health procedures. Women often choose to have their pap smears done by female doctors. Anyone who's had an uncomfortable pap test knows some skill is involved in this procedure and that it takes more time than a standard consultation—but Medicare pays no more for a pap test than a standard consultation.

The insertion of an IUD is another complex procedure that requires additional training to perform. Medicare values this delicate procedure at $53.55. For the insertion of a subcutaneous contraceptive device, such as an Implanon, Medicare pays $35.60. Compare this to the removal and suture of a lesion, which involves some surgical skills more male doctors tend to have than female; for that, Medicare will pay $214.55.

In 2018 the journalist Casey Johnston wrote an excoriating essay that describes the pain of her IUD insertion, and highlights the disparity between how the procedure is downplayed by the medical profession and the steps it involves. Johnston wrote:

> IUD insertion is at least as likely as not to be the worst pain you've ever felt, with virtually no options for recourse or relief. If men were routinely faced with this scenario they would riot in the streets. Some of this appears to vary based on things like cervix position—if it's not pointed directly at the back of your uterus, the doctor has to steer it around and set it in position before they can put the IUD in place. Picture one of those plastic water bottles (this is a uterus) with one of those sport nozzles (this is a cervix) and now squish that nozzle in and crank it to one side. This is how a cervix can be, but it has to be set into a straight position temporarily in order to insert an IUD. It also depends how dilated your cervix might already be; some doctors will advise you to try and have your insertion during your period, when you might be ever so slightly dilated already, to save a couple

millimeters of wrenching you open. Some doctors will give women a mifepristone pill the day before, which dilates you a bit; some will tell you to take some Advil beforehand. Some will put numbing gel on your cervix.

Even under ideal anatomical conditions, there is still likely to be pain but doctors provide no post-op pain medication other than one over-the-counter pill, no Vicodin, no codeine.[40]

Another journalist reported: 'My IUD insertion experience was a debacle of the highest order.'[41] Yet another described her experience as 'pain on a cosmic level'.[42]

I've had a Mirena put in, and I don't think these women are exaggerating, though not all women experience such debilitating pain. I know how long it takes and how painful it can be, and so I know the level of skill needed for the doctor to do it well. A nurse is required to set up the treatment room for the procedure, and in my case was present throughout.

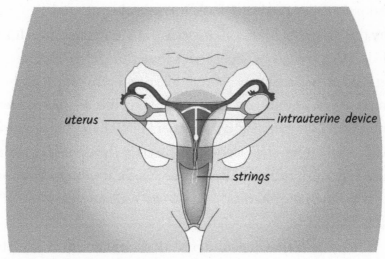

Fitting an IUD through the cervix can be painful.

I'm shocked and horrified to learn those two professionals earned the princely sum of $53.55 between them: the practice has to pay both staff members out of that fee. Now I understand why it wasn't bulk-billed, and I have no regret in paying the gap. Why shouldn't my GP earn more than that? Her colleagues might have seen three patients in that time. Most consultations are 'standard', lasting less than 20 minutes, for which Medicare pays $37.60, so those colleagues could have earnt up to $112.80 in the time I was having my Mirena put in—more than double the rebate for the device insertion—or they could simply have conducted one 'long' consultation for which Medicare pays $72.80. I don't blame GPs who choose not to gain the extra accreditation required to perform this procedure. Where's the incentive for it?

'There's a real dichotomy there between women's work and men's work in medicine,' Dr Anita Saldanha tells me. Saldanha is calm but forthright, coming across as someone who cares very much about people but doesn't suffer fools. She's exactly the kind of personality I look for in a doctor, and I can see why the so-called heartsink patients are attracted to her. It isn't softness that creates her appeal, it's something else—something that makes her seem in charge, alert and eminently capable; someone you could trust to sort out your life. Female patients with borderline personality disorder, PTSD and chronic pain flock to Saldanha; she's known in town as the doctor to see for those types of problems. But while Medicare does allow, and pay for, long consultations, this doesn't always add up to fair compensation.

'They say, "Oh, equal hours work should be equal pay", but it's not because it's fee for service. We don't get paid equally.

And patients self-select. I can't say I'm not going to see 20-
to 40-year-old women. Except some men seem to get away
with basically doing that. A [male colleague] has done no pap
smears in his career. I did four yesterday. In a day. I don't mind
doing pap smears, it doesn't bother me. I just get cross about
the fact that there's no recognition it is a specialised skill.' She
talks about the severe PTSD patient she saw the day before,
which took a long time, and says her male colleague did four
excisions—which Medicare rewards highly—in the time it
took her to see one patient. These are some of the reasons
there's a pay gap in general practice, Saldanha says.

Clare Fairweather runs a general practice in Adelaide
dedicated to treating endometriosis and chronic pelvic pain
conditions. This is a boon to South Australian women because
GPs—and gynaecologists—au fait with the condition and the
latest best-practice treatment are hard to come by. The current
Medicare model is most definitely not supportive of treating
patients with endometriosis, chronic pelvic pain and other
complex conditions, well, Fairweather tells me. Her initial
consultations go something like this:

'I will do a 45 minute to an hour assessment with them
to try and get an understanding about all of the pains that
they're having. So it's not just about their periods . . . I ask
very specific questions about their gut, about the bowel,
about the bladder, the vulval skin, about sexual pain, about
musco-skeletal pain, very specific questions about headaches,
very specific questions about pain generally and some other
symptoms that many of these women all seem to have. They're
all fainty, sickey, nauseated. They often have a very disordered
temperature regulation, and fatigue—the intense fatigue that

goes with this. So when I first start working with them, I'll do a big assessment of how we're going with all of these things. And the mood, of course, is also an extremely important thing to assess and address.'

Medicare in Australia and the National Health Service in England both have programs to manage patients with chronic diseases. In the UK, endo sufferers are eligible to sign up to the Expert Patient Program for the management of chronic disease. In Australia, Medicare offers incentives for GPs to manage their patients with long-term complex diseases under a chronic disease management plan or team care arrangement. The definition of a chronic disease is any condition that 'has been (or is likely to be) present for six months or longer'. The diagnosis is at the GP's discretion, and a 2018 study published in *Australian Health Review* found that endo fits the definition of chronic disease, and should be reclassified as such in clinical practice guidelines and consensus statements; the study concludes that this approach would benefit patients.[43]

This is exactly the approach that Fairweather takes with her endo and chronic pelvic pain patients. 'Unfortunately,' she says, 'a lot of GPs are still stuck in the idea that it's got to be heart disease or diabetes and that nothing else qualifies [for the chronic disease management program]. That is not the case.' Fairweather usually works with physiotherapists, pain psychologists and dieticians, and she says they're helpful for women with pelvic pain. But she says even the additional money Medicare provides for these management plans doesn't always add up to adequate compensation for the work involved: 'Because I spend a lot of time at meetings with my pelvic pain colleagues, then a lot of time doing emails backwards and forwards, I spend a lot of time on the phone, so in fact it's not brilliantly remunerated . . . The complexity of endo in particular means that for many of these women, you will be seeing them a lot, because they have a lot of pain, they need a lot of support. You have to do a lot of walking along-side, because I can't actually fix their pain a lot of the time so I need to be available.'

Now let's take a quick look at gynaecology to see how complex women's health problems are undervalued. Dr Susan Evans sums up the dilemma. 'Basically, a gynaecolo-gist, for example, or a GP that sees a pelvic pain patient, is losing money on every patient. Medicare does not rebate it.' In trying to understand this better, Evans conducted an analysis of Medicare item numbers. Gynaecologists receive $72.50 for a consultation, which may take up to an hour if, as Fair-weather does, the doctor is to gain a full picture of all the pain and complications experienced by chronic pain conditions. But most gynaecologists don't see their job as addressing all the myriad symptoms of a condition—they're paid to operate. Gynaecologists just aren't paid to manage chronic pain. And because they focus on the reproductive organs, their patients may not report many symptoms that seem unrelated, such as headaches, dizziness, fatigue and anxiety, and gynaecologists often either don't ask about or skip over these symptoms, not believing they can help.

Evans' analysis is supported by Young's research in Australia and by the UK's All-Party Parliamentary Group (APPG) on Women's Health inquiry into endometriosis and fibroids, which both show that gynaecologists see their jobs as surgeons who cut things out and not as doctors who manage chronic pain.

This has created a situation in which endo sufferers are having multiple surgeries, often every two years, to remove lesions with little to no benefit. But Fairweather, Evans and other leading gynaecologists—including Dr Jason Abbott, a professor of gynaecological surgery at the University of New South Wales and medical director of Endometriosis Australia—believe this is the wrong approach. They all say one or two high-quality operations conducted by a doctor skilled in laparoscopic excision surgery and with a specialised knowledge of endo should be sufficient for managing the physical disease and adhesions within the pelvic cavity.

In early 2018, following the news of the US actress Lena Dunham's hysterectomy, I commissioned Abbott to write for *The Guardian* about why multiple surgeries often aren't the best treatment for women and others with a uterus who have endo. Dunham had ten laparoscopic surgeries to remove endo with no pain relief, before finally opting to have her uterus surgically removed. While a hysterectomy often doesn't cure the pain of endo, Dunham had other uterine problems that this surgery was intended to help with. Undergoing ten surgeries for endo isn't an uncommon experience in Australia, but Abbott explained that greater numbers of surgeries 'may actually *increase* pain'. He wrote: 'For some endometriosis sufferers undergoing surgery, there is limited or even no response and if there is recurrence of pain symptoms within a few months or even a year, then repeat surgery is probably not going to provide a better outcome for them.'[44]

Many sufferers believe that when pain returns after surgery, it's because the endo has grown back. But this isn't always the case: researchers now understand that endo is a chronic inflammatory condition, and that much of the pain and other symptoms aren't about the physical disease but are the result of central sensitisation (which is described in the next chapter). Fairweather calls endometriosis a 'pain syndrome' and says explaining how pain works to her patients is a vital part of her care. 'I try hard to move people away from that really biologically driven idea that there is abnormal tissue in the pelvis and it just needs to be cut out.' It's not helpful, she says, because it's this idea that drives patients to return for operation after operation. 'I spend quite a lot of time with them explaining the pain, and explaining that endo does seem to trigger off all these pain syndromes, and just because you've got a really dodgy bladder, doesn't mean that you've got endo all over your bladder—you might have—but even if you haven't at laparoscopy, it doesn't mean that you don't have problems with your bladder that are a pain syndrome that's been unmasked, if you like, by the endo.'

Evans says that patients often return to have surgery for pain that's actually caused by muscle spasms in the pelvic region, rather than endometriosis cysts or lesions. She too believes many of the symptoms related to endo and other chronic pelvic pain conditions aren't the result of endometrial tissue, and that repeated surgeries could worsen the pain. But there is no incentive in Australia or the UK for gynaecologists to manage chronic pelvic pain.

'Any gynaecologist that only does pelvic pain, does it well and doesn't do many laparoscopies, can't afford to stay open . . . There's an underlying disincentive to offer anything apart from surgery and hormones,' Evans says. And here again, Medicare and other healthcare systems work against good results, with no distinction between basic ablation surgery, where lesions are simply lasered off, and highly complex excision surgery by an experienced surgeon trained to look for the varied ways endo presents inside the body. 'It actually takes a lot more work, a lot more training, a lot more effort and it's a lot more stressful to do a proper excision than to zap a few things. So doing a laparoscopy where you're there, you zap a few things and you don't do anything that looks tricky, still basically does get you the same pay [as skilled excision surgery].'

The *Pelvic Pain Report*, endorsed by Pain Australia and the Faculty of Pain Medicine Australia and New Zealand, acknowledges the challenges facing gynaecologists in treating chronic pelvic pain, including that this pain isn't recognised as a valid clinical entity. There's currently no viable career structure for Australian gynaecologists wishing to improve their skills managing pelvic pain and no incentives for them to manage chronic pelvic pain (CPP). In consultation on the report, the Royal Australian and New Zealand College of Obstetricians and Gynaecologists raised the issue of the public health coding system for pelvic pain, which hinders data gathering, stifles accurate research and skews funding allocation requirements. They also raised the issue of remuneration, which is based on patient throughput rather than the complexity of conditions with which patients present. The report concludes: 'A change in the Medicare rebate is required to overcome this barrier. There is currently no incentive to manage CPP patients efficiently and effectively because of the complex nature of these conditions.'[45]

The UK's APPG report presented very similar findings. While the United Kingdom has a sophisticated network of specialist endometriosis centres that have proven success rates, they mainly treat deep-infiltrating endo—just one subtype of the disease. Women in the UK face similar long delays in diagnosis to those in Australia, and similar problems finding doctors equipped to deal with their varied and complex complaints. Gynaecologists are encouraged only to operate and there is very little support in the NHS for GPs to prescribe all the various therapies needed by a chronic pain patient.

Young argues a fundamental change is required to how healthcare works in most industrialised nations. 'Our health-care system, and also how medical knowledge works, just has not really been set up for chronic disease, it's been set up very much for acute episodes. If something very clear is wrong, we fix it, then that patient goes away.' She says the health-care system isn't set up for—and doctors aren't trained to deal with—patients who keep coming back with symptoms that can't be cured. 'Someone coming back again and again asking for help to manage their condition, that again poses another challenge to medical knowledge and authority.' She lists chronic fatigue syndrome and fibromyalgia as well as endometriosis as examples of where this most tellingly plays out—all conditions mainly diagnosed in and experienced by women.

The World Health Organization warns that the global burden of chronic disease is increasing rapidly. It's clear we need an urgent strategy to address the ways these patients are cared for. Chronic disease currently represents a huge cost burden on healthcare systems worldwide, but evidence suggests it isn't being treated in a cost-effective manner; repeated surgeries for endometriosis when pelvic physiotherapy could be more effective is just one example, and there's increasing evidence that physiotherapy is more effective—and cheaper—than surgical interventions in treating pelvic organ prolapse and incontinence. Early intervention, education and prevention strategies are essential to treating chronic disease more effectively—but these services are not currently incentivised in our health systems. For my pain, pelvic physiotherapy has been just as effective as surgery, and yet pelvic physios are rare and expensive. On the other hand, the extremely inexpensive drug amitriptyline (it costs me less than $10 for two months' supply) has been hugely effective in treating my pain and improving my quality of life but I was not prescribed this by my GP or gynaecologist—both of whom I rate very highly. I only got a prescription after I discovered the drug while researching this book. Many doctors are still failing to see endometriosis or chronic pelvic pain as a chronic pain condition worthy of any intervention other than surgery or hormones.

As it stands, the system is stacked against the complex needs of women and others with female reproductive systems. But, as Young says, managing complex patients isn't as difficult as some people make out, even when there's a knowledge gap in the disease and a lack of evidence for effective treatments. 'Do you need evidence to provide quality healthcare that recognises your patient's full humanity?' Young says to me. 'I think you can still provide care that addresses people's needs even without research evidence. Medicine has become so equated with science that we've forgotten about the art part of it, or the bedside manner part of it.'

'I JUST WISH DOCTORS KNEW TO LISTEN'

Doctors should listen to their patients. This may sound obvious, but Young's research has found that many doctors discount or dismiss women's reports of their diseases, or treat them with suspicion. Some doctors told Young that they believed they had to confirm women's stories themselves, or believed they'd be able to tell whether the patient's reports were true or not. 'Women's knowledge was typically incorporated only once it had been filtered through the medical gaze, with clinicians extracting what they deemed relevant.'[46] How doctors think they can work this out in a single 20-minute (or shorter) consultation was never explained. As bizarre as this sounds, it's widespread practice. Doctors are, in their own and society's eyes, the ultimate judges of who is sick and who is 'crazy'.

This issue rose to prominence during the women's health movements of the 1970s, spurred along by women such as Harvard Medical School's first female dean, Dr Mary C. Howell. In a 1974 report for the *New England Journal of Medicine*, she wrote:

Following traditional linguistic convention, patients in most medical-school lectures are referred to exclusively by the male pronoun, 'he'. There is, however, a notable exception: in discussing a hypothetical patient whose disease is of psychogenic origin, the lecturer often automatically uses 'she'. For it is widely taught, both explicitly and implicitly, that women patients (when they receive notice at all) have uninteresting illnesses, are unreliable historians, and are beset by such emotionality that their symptoms are unlikely to reflect 'real' disease.[47]

It would be comforting to think that a lot has changed since the awareness-raising heyday of the 1970s—but today's prevalence of medically unexplained symptoms (MUS) is evidence that it has not. The UK National Health Service lists being a woman as the major risk factor of being diagnosed with MUS, and the circular logic and potential for harm in a diagnosis of these symptoms is infuriating. If an illness is hard to diagnose, it often gets dumped into the MUS basket, which makes other doctors less likely to keep searching for a diagnosis and far less likely to trust the patient, even if they seek help for an entirely different issue.

In *Doing Harm*, Maya Dusenbery calls this the double bind of medicine's knowledge and trust gap: 'Women's symptoms are not taken seriously because medicine doesn't know as much about their bodies and health problems. And medicine doesn't know as much about their bodies and health problems because it doesn't take their symptoms seriously.'[48] Having a diagnosis of MUS or anxiety makes it much harder for a patient to be taken seriously by any health professional, as almost any symptom they present with can be shrugged off as anxiety or stress. In her 1978 book *Illness as Metaphor*, Susan Sontag wrote: 'Theories that diseases are caused by mental states and can be cured by will power are always an index of how much is not understood about the physical terrain of a disease.'[49]

In cases where a physical disease is present but can't be controlled, medicine tends to position it as 'uniquely mysterious and by finding fault within the women who experience it'.[50] But actually listening to sufferers may be the act of demystification that allows for better treatment and sharper research focus.

Evans is a great advocate of listening. In her eighteen years of treating women with pelvic pain, she has asked them to record their symptoms in questionnaires. From this data she has established that women with severe period pain (with or without endometriosis) usually have a combination of fourteen symptoms in addition to their severe dysmenorrhea, which include: stabbing pains in the pelvis, bowel problems, food intolerances, bladder problems, headaches, sexual pain, vulval pain, fatigue, poor sleep, nausea, sweating, dizziness/faint, anxiety and low mood.

Evans published a study in the *Journal of Pain Research* showing that women with severe period pain, on average, have eight-and-a-half other symptoms from that pool of fourteen.[51] This study didn't take place in a lab. By listening to, believing, recording and analysing women's reports of their illnesses, Evans now understands a lot more about endo and other forms of pelvic pain—which is informing her research today.

One patient who contributed to the UK APPG inquiry into endometriosis and fibroids said, 'I just wish doctors knew to LISTEN, we know our bodies better than anyone else.'[52] The inquiry's report noted: 'Of the over 1000 plus comments that we received for endometriosis almost every person spoke about being dismissed by healthcare professionals and having to fight for a diagnosis, information and treatment.'[53]

Evans says, 'I have loads of people who come along and say, "My GP says I'm a mystery and that they don't know what's happening". And I think, "Your story's exactly the same as the last person I saw. It's no mystery."'

It struck me when Evans used these words that I'd heard an almost identical sentiment out of the mouth of Dr Nikki Stamp, one of fewer than twelve female cardiothoracic surgeons in Australia. Stamp, who's based in Perth, has written a book on heart disease and is an energetic campaigner for greater understanding of this disease in women. She sighs over the phone when I speak to her, telling me about how often women's heart disease symptoms are misdiagnosed as anxiety. 'It happens all the time,' she says, before sharing the story of a women in her 40s who'd just had a heart attack. The patient had presented to her GP and to emergency departments several times with symptoms including shortness of breath and discomfort in her chest, but was diagnosed with anxiety and sent home. 'She finally got admitted to hospital and someone finally thought to check out her heart, fully expecting to find nothing actually but ended up finding something quite serious. She had a blockage in one of her major arteries in her heart. It's a blockage we tend to refer to as a "widow maker", it's that serious that traditionally it's been associated with people just dropping dead,' Stamp says. 'It's always the same story when you hear about a patient like this.' She says the male doctors always sit around saying things like, 'Wow, this is really unusual, how amazing, never would have seen that coming.' In her exasperation, she is sometimes accused of jumping on a feminist soapbox when she points out, 'But we do see these stories all the time. It's not unusual, it's not uncommon, it's not amazing. Why are we accepting this as such an anomaly? Why aren't we thinking about this as the norm?'

Because the norm in heart disease is a 70-kilogram white man, that's why. And even though the research on the differences in heart disease and presentations of heart attacks in men and women is out there and accepted, says Stamp, it just won't sink in with some doctors that this female patient's presentation was entirely normal. Not all men have typical symptoms either so more recognition of so-called atypical presentations would ultimately benefit everyone.

After patients are listened to and trusted, treatments often become more effective. In Young's study on endometriosis, one GP reported how her practice had improved when she started asking patients to keep diaries of their symptoms.[54] Fairweather, meanwhile, describes listening to patients as 'the most valuable thing' a doctor has in treating them: 'You've got to listen, you've got to have your ears open and you've got to hear it, don't dismiss it. What is the problem for this person at this time?' She says it's vital to understand the patient's priorities and accept that these may not be yours as a doctor. Women's illnesses become decidedly less mysterious when we really listen to, and believe, what they're saying.

Dr Mona Orady, director of robotic surgery at St Francis Memorial Hospital in San Francisco, practises minimally invasive gynaecological surgery at Dignity Medical Foundation. Her expertise is in complex surgery, menstrual disorders, fibroids and endometriosis. She also cares for more specialised gynae-cology patients with pelvic pain, dyspareunia, vulvar disorders and paediatric gynaecological conditions. She says she treats 'the problem, not the pathology'. 'We have to FIFE patients,' she says. 'What FIFE stands for is we have to ask patients about their feelings, their ideas, their fears and their expectations.' She says she asks every patient what their goals are, and what they want to achieve by seeing her, before she can decide what level of treatment should get them back to their normal life. 'I can't just treat the disease, I have to treat how it impacts their life.'

In his 2007 book, *How Doctors Think*, Jerome Groopman interviews Debra Roter, a professor of health policy and management at Johns Hopkins University, about how doctors diagnose patients. 'The doctor has to make the patient feel that he is really interested in hearing in what they have to say. And when a patient tells his story, the patient gives cue and clues to what the doctor may not be thinking.'[55] Another doctor, Sir William Osler—who, when he died in 1919, was 'widely judged to have been among the greatest physicians of all time'[56]—became famous for teaching, 'Just listen to your patient, he is telling you the diagnosis.'[57] The problem is, listening to 'him' has never extended to listening to 'her'.

The idea of listening sounds so basic, yet when it comes to women, it seems it's not so basic at all. This isn't unique to medicine: society at large has a problem with listening to, and believing, women—this is what the #MeToo movement is essentially about.

And as Maya Dusenbery acknowledges, there's always a gap between when symptoms emerge and when they can be medically explained:

> It is unreasonable to expect that doctors, who are fallible human beings doing a difficult job, can close this gap instantaneously—and, given that medical knowledge is, and probably always will be, incomplete, they may at times not be able to close it at all. But it shouldn't be unreasonable to expect that, during this period of uncertainty, the benefit of the doubt be given to the patient, the default assumption be that their symptoms are real, their description of what they are feeling in their own bodies be believed, and, if it is 'medically unexplained', the burden be on medicine to explain it. Such basic trust has been denied to women for far too long.[58]

I've been on the receiving end of this distrust since my teenage years. But while writing this book, I had another alarming experience. I had crippling abdominal pain and constipation that lasted three days—it was a pain I'd never felt before, and I could barely move. I was nauseated and feverish.

After the third night with little sleep, I went to the emergency room at the local hospital. I'd only been to an emergency department two other times: once in India after being run over by a train, and another time in Australia after having concurrent vomiting and diarrhoea for 12 hours because of food poisoning. I'd never been for pain.

Because my partner had worked in emergency departments for years, I was familiar with the in-jokes about patients rocking up at midnight with a sore back they'd had for six months. I knew that 'go see your GP in the morning' is the war cry of emergency physicians who are constantly under pressure and annoyed by people who fail to understand the meaning of 'emergency'. But my partner, who was out of town, knew this pain was unusual and suggested I needed a physical examination. I was temporarily living an hour's drive from my excellent GP, so I drove the 10 minutes around to the hospital just before 6 am.

The nurses who greeted me were pleasant, and there were no other patients in the waiting room. An intern came to see me, listened to my symptoms, ordered an X-ray and asked me to lie on the examination table. Then I told her about my endo and how I'd had it removed from my bowel a few years earlier. I thought that giving all the information I had, anything that might be relevant, would be helpful.

The intern left the room to speak to the consultant.

She came back a few minutes later and said I should see my gynaecologist because 'this sounds like endometriosis'.

I explained calmly that I couldn't just pop in to see my gynaecologist when I wasn't feeling well. And I'd had endometriosis my entire adult life—in 20 years of pain, I'd never gone to an emergency department. 'I know what my endometriosis pain feels like,' I said. 'I know how to manage that pain. This pain is different, I'm worried about it. You haven't even done a physical exam. I just want to know there's nothing serious happening with my bowel!'

She perfunctorily prodded my stomach for a few seconds, then said she'd get the consultant to talk to me directly. But she came back without him and handed me a referral to a private diagnostic imaging clinic for an abdominal ultrasound to rule out appendicitis, cholelithiasis and renal tract obstruction—all serious conditions that if genuinely suspected would have to be treated immediately, and so should have been ruled out in the emergency department.

'I'm not an idiot,' I said to her. 'I know what's happening here. You hear endometriosis and you think I'm either hysterical or a hypochondriac.' The intern blushed. I walked out, and cried all the way to my GP's surgery, stopping regularly to hunch over in pain or wait for the nausea and dizzy spells to pass.

It turned out I had a gastro virus, and under my GP's care I felt better within a couple of days. But I'd been treated like a fool, dismissed, ignored and humiliated. I actually felt ashamed that it was only a virus, not an emergency after all; maybe the consultant had been right not to see me, and I'd just been worked up because I hadn't slept properly in three days and had taken a lot painkillers—had I taken too many?

I was diagnosing myself with hysteria, ashamed and embarrassed at my behaviour. But when I told my partner what had happened, he was incensed. The ultrasound referral was confirmation of my suspicion the consultant had written me off as a hypochondriac without even speaking to me face to face. In giving all the information I had about my health, I thought I was being helpful but to the emergency consultant, it translated as me being a highly strung woman anxious about my health. I've been asked by doctors before, 'Are you often anxious about your health?' and I know at this point they're writing me off as a 'somatiser' or hypochondriac, someone with nothing better to do than pester doctors over trivial concerns. But my partner said the consultant's response was unethical, sloppy work, and that it could lead to people dying. And the statistics back him up.

In 2016, *The BMJ* reported that medical errors in general are the third leading cause of death in the United States, after heart disease and cancer.[59] In Australia, by some estimates, as many as 18,000 people die every year as a result of medical error. About 50,000 suffer a permanent injury. One in six patients in the UK is misdiagnosed. These figures are conservative because currently there isn't an efficient way to collect data about misdiagnoses and medical errors, but they're widely acknowledged as a problem. A WHO report found that misdiagnoses were most often the result of a problem in the clinical encounter between doctor and patient, with failing to take a proper history—medical terminology for asking the patient questions and making decisions based on the answers—one of the major factors involved.

In his book, Groopman tells the story of a young woman

with irritable bowel syndrome who nearly died of a ruptured ectopic pregnancy after being dismissed by three doctors when she reported abdominal pain that was different from her usual IBS pain.[60] A nurse I spoke to recently told a remarkably similar story of being ignored and having her pain dismissed by doctors until she was diagnosed with an ectopic pregnancy.

These stories aren't rare, and in September 2018, covering a coronial inquest for *The Guardian*, I was faced with the truth of this. As well as another painful truth on top of it: however bad I felt for not being believed, for Australian Aboriginal women it is much, much worse, and the consequences are deadly.

DISADVANTAGED WOMEN

The inquest I sat in on was looking into the death of Naomi Williams, a 27-year-old Wiradjuri woman who was six months pregnant at the time of her death. The facts are taken from the evidence at the inquest. She died from a sepsis associated with the bacterium *Neisseria meningitidis*—a serious but treatable infection—15 hours after being discharged from the emergency department of her local hospital. The inquest was concerned not with the cause of death but with the treatment Naomi had received from the hospital in the six months leading up to her death—and whether that treatment was a factor in it.

Naomi was described as a joyful woman with lots of friends and close family, and she'd won awards for her work in adult disability support. 'She was a very caring person,' her mother, Sharon Williams, told my colleague at *The Guardian*, Melissa Davey. 'She was very proud of her [Wiradjuri] culture and her identity. She was loved by everyone she worked with and by her community. We used to call her Miss Chatterbox because she was always talking to everyone, and she would have done anything for anyone.'[61]

Australians have a long life expectancy—we rank fifth in the OECD at an average of 82.5 for both men and women, staying at fifth for men but moving down to eighth place for women. But Aboriginal and Torres Strait Islander people live an average of ten fewer years than their non-Indigenous compatriots. An Australian Aboriginal girl born in 2018 is expected to live to be 73.7 while non-Indigenous Australian women can expect to live until the ripe old age of 83.1.[62] Maternal and child mortality rates are also worse among Aboriginal and Torres Strait Islander women than other Australians: the mortality rate for Indigenous infants was 5.0 deaths per 1000 live births in 2012, compared to 3.3 for non-Indigenous infants. Still, this is an improvement since 1998, when it was 13.5 for Indigenous infants and 4.4 for non-Indigenous infants. The maternal mortality rate for Indigenous women is more than double that for other Australian women.[63]

In 2015, Naomi Williams became ill with chronic stomach pain, nausea and frequent episodes of vomiting and diarrhoea. She went to the hospital's emergency department eighteen different times—and to medical centres many more times—with these symptoms. Two years earlier she'd had her gall bladder removed and was worried the symptoms could be related.

But at the hospital, Naomi was usually sent home after receiving some medication to stop the vomiting and IV fluids to treat dehydration. She was referred at least three times to drug-and-alcohol and mental health services, even though their assessments consistently showed no drug or alcohol abuse problems and no mental health issues. She was never referred to a specialist for investigation of her pain symptoms.

Eventually, Naomi did develop some anxiety and depression associated with not having her pain treated and not being believed by medical staff. She began to think the staff had stigmatised her as a drug addict and wouldn't take her symptoms seriously.

Naomi was right: doctors and nursing staff had decided her nausea was down to marijuana use, since she'd admitted to occasionally smoking the drug in order to ease her pain and help her sleep. In coronial evidence from Naomi's partner, Michael Lampe, and her cousin, Talea Bulger, the court heard that Naomi hated going to the hospital when ill, became anxious when admitted and almost never went alone for fear of how the staff would treat her. On one occasion, when attending the hospital with Naomi, Talea heard a nurse comment, 'Oh, you're back again.'

Naomi became so upset by her treatment at the hospital, her mother wrote to its health services manager begging her to refer Naomi to a specialist and to stop referring her to drug-and-alcohol services. She explained the only cause of Naomi's mental health problems was being stereotyped as a drug addict and not having her pain taken seriously.

'There are problems in Tumut with people abusing prescription drugs, and people seeking out the drugs from hospitals, and I feel as though Naomi was tarred with the same brush,' Sharon Williams told my colleague Davey. 'I honestly think that's why they referred her to drug and mental health services. But she was a hard worker, the kind of person who hated to let anyone down. She didn't have drug or mental health problems. But she was sick, and in pain.'[64]

The next time Naomi visited the hospital she was pregnant, and the referral to a specialist never came. Once again, the only referral she received was to drug-and-alcohol services. Since she was now pregnant, Naomi's pain and vomiting symptoms were diagnosed as hyperemesis gravidarum, a severe form of morning sickness. The symptoms persisted through her pregnancy, and she was admitted to another hospital in the nearest capital city after an urgent referral from her GP.

On the day before Naomi died, Michael and Talea reported, she was feeling very sick. According to Michael, who was caring for his young daughter that night as well, Naomi had gone to bed around eight-thirty after vomiting and complaining of a headache, back pain and spasms. At around midnight, Michael urged her to go to the hospital. Feeling too sick to drive, she texted Talea: 'You wouldn't be able to get me to hospital, would you? I can barely move.' But Talea was at a New Year's Eve party and didn't get the message, so Naomi ended up driving herself.

The nurses' testimony in court contradicted Michael's and Talea's accounts. They described Naomi as looking like she was 'blossoming' from pregnancy and said she only came to hospital to ask for two paracetamol as she had none at home, a claim Michael denied.[65]

Naomi was in the hospital for 34 minutes before being discharged by nurses. No formal pain assessment was taken, no history, no physical examination—even though she was six months pregnant, had been admitted to another hospital recently and was complaining of hip pain relating to the pregnancy. And no doctor was called to see her. At the inquest, the nurses said Naomi had denied vomiting that evening, telling them she hadn't thrown up for two days, and they claimed she hadn't mentioned the headaches or spasms Michael said she'd been complaining of. Asked how to explain why Naomi was sucking a Hydralyte iceblock, a common treatment for nausea and dehydration, when she arrived at the hospital, one of the nurses said, 'I don't know, she just liked to eat ice.' Sepsis is more common in pregnant women and in Aboriginal people than the rest of the population, and Australian medical staff are trained to be more suspicious of sepsis in these cases.

Fifteen hours after the hospital staff gave Naomi two paracetamol and sent her home, she was dead. She died in an ambulance on the way back to hospital, after delaying going for hours because of fear she wouldn't be believed.

Sepsis can be hard to diagnose in its early stages, but would the nurses have asked more questions, kept her in longer for observation and completed a physical examination if Naomi had been white? Would she have spoken up more forcefully about her symptoms if she hadn't suspected the nurses thought she was an addict? Would she have returned to the hospital earlier as her condition dramatically deteriorated if she hadn't been sent home so dismissively only hours before? These are the questions the NSW deputy coroner, Harriet Grahame, will be trying to answer in her final report, which had not yet been handed down when this book went to print. Her findings will hopefully inform health policy and training in Australia, and challenge the way Aboriginal women are treated in our healthcare system.

Naomi had planned to move to Canberra, where her mother lived and where she was confident of receiving better care, to give birth. She'd booked in with an Aboriginal health service to have her baby, and her mother had planned to retire so she could help with the care. Naomi and Michael were excited about the birth of their son; they had dreams and hopes and plans. But Naomi was cursed with chronic pain symptoms that doctors decided were due to drug use, and not worth referral to a specialist. She faced so many challenges: being a woman and having symptoms that doctors can't explain is itself a huge barrier to good treatment. But on top of that, Naomi faced entrenched racism and stereotypes about Aboriginal and black people that contaminate the Western world.

In 2016, an American study found that black patients were half as likely to be prescribed opioid drugs in emergency departments for non-definitive pain than white patients.[66] It has long been suspected that people of colour are treated negatively by doctors partly because of prejudiced misconceptions about biological differences between black and white people. Another 2016 study found that a substantial number of white medical students and registrars believed false stereotypes that black people have thicker skin than white people, their nerve endings are less sensitive, and that their blood coagulates more quickly than white people's.[67] 'Black patients are not afforded the luxury of being seen in EDs, physician offices, and clinics as just patients in need of help and healing,' said Keisha Ray, a postdoctoral fellow with the McGovern Center for Humanities and Ethics at the University of Texas Health Science Center at Houston. She added, 'Rather they are seen as less than human, drug seekers and overall exaggerators.'[68]

Rebecca Manson Jones, health spokesperson for the UK Women's Equality Party, tells me this is also the case in the UK: 'We know anecdotally and we know from all the evidence that women who have any form of . . . minority [status] are less likely to take advantage of the health service, for a number of different reasons. Whether it's cultural or financial or because their expectation is that they won't get good service.'

Unfortunately their expectation is all too often correct.

CHAPTER 6

'The pain that can't be seen': a new appreciation of women's pain

One of my earliest memories is of pain. I don't know my exact age but I can't have been older than three or four, jumping on a trampoline with a little girl my age; our mothers were sitting in the kitchen having a cup of tea. In those days, trampolines weren't surrounded by nets and their springs weren't padded. I jumped and jumped, ever higher, until I lost my footing and my leg slipped through a gap between the mat and steel structure, and my thigh became enmeshed in a spring.

I screamed. We had a large backyard and my mum didn't hear, but my friend ran up to the house, I assumed to get her attention. Trapped, I sat there crying, waiting for my mum to fix it all, like she always did. But my little friend didn't alert the grown-ups, and I remember a feeling of loneliness and betrayal as I sat there, overwhelmed by pain and disbelief.

Over the next few years, I sprained an ankle jumping off a rock at the beach, tore a ligament in my knee with more trampoline antics, and broke my pinky finger playing basketball. I tried to explain the pain to my mum: 'It feels like the ache in this little finger is radiating through my entire body!' She gave me a look that was mostly sympathetic but also a little amused.

After that came menstrual issues: the cramps, the diarrhoea, the back pain, that sharp ache that felt like a rod down the front of my right leg, the heavy, *heavy* legs, the agony, the sheer exhaustion of it all, too often huddled over and walking through thick sludge. It got worse, year after year, until I became a regular in the school sick bay and Mum knew to expect a call once a month. No one ever supposed there was something wrong with me. It was period pain—wasn't that normal?

Eventually my mum took me to a new doctor, who referred me to an immunologist, who diagnosed me with chronic fatigue syndrome. I was treated with gamma globulin injections—which is a blood plasma product—since the doctor felt my white blood cell count was low. I felt a little better for a while after that but still have vivid memories of period pain, of begging my mum for pain relief and lying on the floor with my legs up the wall to ease the pain. This was just a feature of my life.

At nineteen, I went skiing for the first time. I was young, fearless . . . and stupid. I lost a ski coming off a small jump and slammed my back into a large rock. I saw the world upside down, a tree beneath me, looking on the snow from up high as I somersaulted to the ground. I was terrified that I would die or be paralysed when I hit it. And then I did. With a thud. I concentrated on feeling my feet. Yes, I could feel them. I wiggled my toes—I'd seen the movies. But then I realised I was really hurt, and lay still. There was no one around; I was the only one silly enough to try the jump on a sunny day under icy snow.

Then a tourist appeared, peering over me, asking questions in a language I didn't understand. He looked scared, and when he started yelling 'HELP!' at the chairlift and waving his ski poles around frantically, I was relieved, believing that help would soon be here and this would all be cleared up.

Red blood was winding a slow path through the white snow, and a crowd soon gathered around me. I could see them all, but I couldn't talk. I answered the paramedics' questions to show I was conscious but quickly worked out that crying, talking or moving in any way made the pain unbearable. The best strategy was to stay as still as possible. I learnt to use my voice in a way that required the least effort, to answer the questions of the kind nurse accompanying me to the medical centre, checking I was conscious.

I remember the voices and noises in the busy medical clinic. I remember not speaking, not asking for help, not having the capacity to think about how long I was left waiting. I remember a doctor seeing me at last, asking how I got the lacerations on my bum. I didn't answer, no longer able to talk, the pain too intense. I didn't know what had happened but I knew this pain wasn't from a cut. I needed the doctor to find out, not to ask me. But she chatted away. 'Where's all this blood coming from if there are no holes in your pants?' She pulled down the outer ski pants. 'I can't find the holes in your pants. Where did you cut yourself?' She pulled down my leggings and knickers. And gasped. She rang a bell and called for morphine, then asked me, 'Why didn't you say anything?' I still couldn't answer.

Lying there over the next couple of hours, I learnt what the sacrum was—it's the triangular bone at the base of the spine above the coccyx. And I learnt the definition of a compound fracture—it's when a broken bone pierces the skin. And that's where all the blood was coming from—a compound fracture of my sacrum.

I was taken by road ambulance to the nearest major hospital, a drive that took over three hours and that had bumps the morphine couldn't disguise. Urgent tests revealed, thank god, that the stray bone hadn't pierced my bowel or any internal organs and that nerve damage appeared to be limited. But the doctors in Canberra had never seen a compound fracture of the sacrum on a young person, and felt surgery was too risky with the bladder and bowel so close and the nerve endings so complicated in that area.

So I was taken by air ambulance to Sydney, and the morphine was once again a poor competitor to the turbulence. There was a man on that flight who held my hand and told me stories and I felt that I loved him but even he couldn't take away the pain.

In hospital in Sydney, the country's leading orthopaedic surgeons were once again perplexed. Young people don't fracture their sacrum—old ladies with osteoporosis do, and occasionally horseriders. But a healthy nineteen year old, skiing? Unheard of! It was decided that surgery was too risky, and likely to be of little use. So bed rest was ordered. And a whole heap of painkillers.

The pain of that accident lasted a long time. Years. And something happened as a result: I put down all my back pain, hip pain, leg pain, shooting pains in my rectum, pins and needles when opening my bowels, muscle spasms in the pelvis, a right glute that never stopped hurting, to this accident.

At 23, I decided my period pain wasn't normal. No one I knew suffered like I did. No painkillers could relieve it. While my female GP had told me for years that, 'Some women just have bad period pain', and that I'd have to learn to deal with it, I insisted at last on a referral to a gynaecologist.

Lucky for me, I lived near a big hospital, and I lucked out on seeing a gynaecologist who knew a lot about endometriosis and was a skilled laparoscopic surgeon. He suspected endo within a few minutes of our chat and booked me in for an operation he told me would cut out the lesions. I researched this thing called endometriosis at the library, on the internet (which was then still pretty new!), and in medical journals and encyclopaedias I found in the offices of the nursing homes where my mother was director of care.

The endometriosis was severe, and what my doctor thought would be a quick laparoscopy turned into a lengthy operation in which he had to make a larger-than-expected cut in my abdomen and call in another surgeon to help. I had deep infiltrating endometriosis, which had fused my uterus to my rectum and ovaries. And I was diagnosed with stage IV endo, the worst category. What was supposed to be day surgery became a five-night stay in hospital. The pain was awful, but my gynaecologist was kind and informative, offering me hope for the future. He told me not to believe people who said endometriosis equalled infertility—but he added that, since endo grows back, I'd have to see him again when I decided I was ready to become pregnant.

I started taking the pill back to back, usually four months in a row, then having a period. This managed the period pain and meant I could schedule it around important events; I coped well enough with that for many years. But I didn't know my bowel problems, pain and food intolerances were related to the endo. I didn't know the back pain that was a constant companion and that sharp ache down the front of my right leg had anything to do with endo. I certainly didn't know my dizzy spells were related. I didn't know the fatigue—that overwhelming fatigue that slammed right into me at the most inconvenient times, and would reveal itself to the world in the shape of vicious cold sores and a thick foggy brain—was related to my endo. I didn't know that constant ache that regularly sat at the base of my gut—not quite cramps, not quite stabbing pain—was related to endo, although I was confused by that pain because it was like I had period pain when I didn't have my period. I didn't talk about it. When and how do you mention pain in the butt, feeling sick after sex, and pain that isn't enough to complain about out loud?

I went to see physiotherapist after physiotherapist and reported a fractured sacrum as the source of my back pain. No one could help.

In my 30s, I accidentally discovered a pelvic physiotherapist who clocked on to the fact that something was very wrong with my pelvic floor muscles and hips. The exercises she gave me produced the greatest relief I'd ever known. But I never thought to mention my endo to her. Because that was all fine now, I thought. I had occasional bouts of self-pity but friends didn't seem to think my suffering was out of proportion to theirs, and I didn't want to be a drag. I started to internalise the pain, to believe I was just weak. I never had the energy that my friends did. I always paid for my occasional energy bursts in a way I didn't see happening to other people.

And then there was the train. On a suburban Mumbai railway platform in 2012 I tried to jump on to a departing train. Instead, I slipped between the train and platform and tumbled down, tossed around like clothes in a washing machine, until—miraculously—I landed flat on my back, under the moving train. The shouts of 'Don't move!' and 'Stay still!' from strangers probably saved my life. I heard these commands from a fog of confusion, not knowing what had happened or where I was. I decided to stay still just in case they were directed at me. I had some impression that I'd fallen.

I watched the train travel over me, about 20 centimetres above my flat, still body, believing I was about to die. How could I possibly survive being underneath a train?

I emerged with a broken shoulder, a sprained ankle, a ligament torn in a finger, and lots of nasty cuts and bruises on my face, elbow, feet, shins and knees. Blood poured off me, and oil, water and filth filled every scrape. As I was lifted from the track and fussed over by caring locals, I surmised death was still a risk factor from infection if I didn't get the wounds clean soon.

The pain was so intense I didn't sleep for almost 70 hours. But I was alive! People in the guesthouse I was staying at were surprised at how well I was taking it. They laughed when I joked, 'What doesn't kill you makes a good story!' But I'd decided on a strategy not to think about the accident. Recalling being under the train made me panic, sweat and doubt that I was alive or that I should be. The injuries hurt, sure, but I didn't feel *bad*.

Surgery to repair my broken shoulder was also painful, but it didn't make me feel *bad* either. What did was a second laparoscopy to remove endometriosis in 2016, the year I found out I had adenomyosis too. After a colonoscopy revealed extensive bowel damage due to endo, a colorectal surgeon teamed up with my gynaecologist for the laparoscopy with the view to performing a bowel resection: a section of damaged bowel is surgically removed, and the remaining bowel is stitched back together. It's a serious operation with some risks involved.

Thankfully, the two remarkable surgeons managed to remove the endo from my bowel without having to do the resection. This was a great outcome, one I had hoped for, and I was so pleased to hear the news when I awoke. There had also been a concern I could lose an ovary, since ultrasounds showed severe damage and a large endometrioma—a type of cyst—inside one of them. But this too was saved.

Endometriosis was removed from my uterus, ovaries, bowel, pelvic side wall, the Pouch of Douglas and utero-sacral ligaments. It was a long, difficult operation, but both surgeons were pleased with the results, and I'm eternally grateful to them for their precision and skill, and the care they always showed me.

One doctor had told me I'd have to have a hysterectomy because of the adenomyosis. Not only had I kept my uterus, but also both ovaries and an intact bowel.

I've felt so much better since the surgery. But the recovery was awful, the pain in my abdomen severe; it felt like my insides were being carved with knives every time I moved. I was sick, too; I vomited from the nausea. The concoctions of drugs I was being served up seemed random and inconsistent. For seven days after the surgery, I felt worse than I'd ever felt in my life and the week after that wasn't much better. Sick, sore, dizzy, faint, miserable. I was pleased the surgery had been so successful but I couldn't feel happy. I faked smiles for visitors because I was convinced I must be exaggerating the pain and nausea, the heaviness of my body, the sense of dread that something very, very bad was happening to me.

Laparoscopic surgery is hailed for being minimally invasive. The surgeon makes three or four incisions in the abdomen, usually small, through which a laparoscope and surgical instruments are inserted. The laparoscope is a sophisticated camera device that allows the surgeons to see inside the abdomen on a screen in the operating theatre without having to fully cut it open. The approach is designed to speed up recovery and is believed to place the smallest possible burden on the patient. But it didn't feel like this to me.

In the days and weeks after the surgery, for the first time I really thought about pain. I'd never before added up all the pain I'd felt in my life. But now I relived every episode, playing it all out in my mind, obsessively. Felt the injuries, over and over. All this pain suddenly accumulated, and like a flooded dam it washed over me. I was heavy from the burden of it. And choked on it. Every vessel felt constricted, harsh, and to breathe, eat, walk, move a limb, roll over in bed, all required effort. I started to see my body as separate, something apart from me, something cruel and devious and punishing. I came to hate my body and all the pain it had caused.

I know about pain, I thought. I've had a broken back, been run over by a train! If anybody knows what ten is on the 1 to 10 pain scale that they ask you about every hour in hospital, it's me! I know what ten is—it's a broken back; it's a broken shoulder, sprained ankle, head injury and bruised hip lying under a train in Mumbai. That's ten! But that pain was focused and intense, and painkillers worked. They gave me relief, even if brief, from the pain and made me happy: grateful to be alive, not paralysed, in possession of all my limbs, able to make jokes and tell good stories. That pain faded, and I felt better.

But this pain—this pain after the laparoscopy and the pain of endometriosis—is nothing like that. This ache, this always-present gnawing, is the pain that makes me feel *bad*. No painkiller puts me in a happy mood with this pain. No bliss overcomes me. No drug can stop the nausea once it arrives. Only stillness helps. But stillness is so hard. I've felt ten, and I can tell you, this pain is worse.

WHAT IS PAIN?

The International Association for the Study of Pain defines it as 'an unpleasant sensory and emotional experience associated with actual or potential tissue damage, or described in terms of such damage'.[1] Traditionally, pain was thought to belong to one of two categories: acute pain, which was associated with injury or tissue damage and usually lasted a short period of time, or stopped when the tissue damage healed, and chronic pain, which was any pain that lasted for more than three months. It's now understood that there are many different types of pain, with different bodily mechanisms involved.

Until recently medical science has focused on acute pain—that's the pain you get from an injury (a broken leg, a cut finger, a ruptured organ) or after surgery—and is fairly good at treating it. Painkillers you can buy at pharmacies and stronger ones prescribed by a doctor are generally pretty good at easing this pain.

Chronic pain is another story: here, medicine itself acknowledges its shortcomings in both knowledge and effective treatments. This has occurred for a number of reasons. Pain was always considered to be a symptom of an underlying disease or injury, even when that initial condition couldn't be located, but researchers have now discovered that pain may be experienced in the absence of any tissue damage or out of all proportion to the original injury, and can cause biological changes in the peripheral and central nervous systems. We are beginning to understand that chronic pain (sometimes called persistent or ongoing pain) is a syndrome involving the central nervous system, in which it 'becomes hypersensitive and overresponsive to stimuli that normally would not be painful—a light touch or a gentle breeze, for example. In a sense, the nervous system of a person with chronic pain becomes "rewired for pain".'[2] This is different to acute pain, meaning it doesn't respond to the same treatments. At least one in five people experience chronic pain and 30 per cent are severely disabled by it.[3]

Only in 2011, however, did the National Academy for Medicine in the United States declare that chronic pain was a disease condition and had to be treated in its own right. At the time, the academy recognised that chronic pain can also 'engender a range of significant psychological and social consequences, such as fear; anger; depression; anxiety; and reduced ability to carry out one's social roles as family member, friend, and employee'.[4] While other national institutes around the world have followed suit, there's still a massive gap between how many people are affected by chronic pain and medicine's ability to treat it. Doctors haven't been adequately trained to treat chronic pain, and the Western medical science tradition of specialities is ill-equipped to deal with it since it involves multiple body systems and functions.

The 2010 Affordable Care Act that established Obamacare in the United States includes a requirement for the Department of Health and Human Services to work with the Institute of Medicine (IOM) 'to increase the recognition of pain as a significant public health problem in the United States'.[5] The IOM was commissioned to conduct a study to assess the state of the science regarding pain research, care and education, and to make recommendations to advance the field. The resulting report, *Relieving Pain in America*, had global impact. It found that about 100 million adult Americans suffered from chronic pain, with an annual national economic cost of between US$560 and $635 billion. It also found that social stigma, uncertain diagnoses, ineffective treatments and inadequate medical knowledge plagued chronic pain patients. The investigating committee wrote that 'addressing the nation's enormous burden of pain will require a cultural transformation in the way pain is understood, assessed, and treated'.[6]

WOMEN IN PAIN

I can't help but wonder if we're in this position because women outnumber men when it comes to chronic pain. There's a two-to-sixfold greater prevalence and greater intensity of chronic pain syndromes in women compared to men.[7] In fact, the International Association for the Study of Pain notes that women generally experience more recurrent, more severe and longer-lasting pain than men. Fibromyalgia, irritable bowel syndrome (IBS), rheumatoid arthritis, osteoarthritis, temporomandibular joint disorder, chronic pelvic pain and migraine headache are all more prevalent in women than men. In headaches, neck, shoulder, knee and back pain, the ratio of women affected to men is 1.5:1. A Dutch study on pain in children showed that the difference in experience of pain between the sexes started from a young age; while in the first three years of life, boys experience marginally more pain than girls, then between four and seven years of age girls start to outnumber boys. Between the ages of eight and eleven, more than double the number of girls than boys experience pain, and the ratio continues to increase from twelve to eighteen years of age. Researchers found that girls were more likely to experience multiple pains and more severe chronic pains.[8]

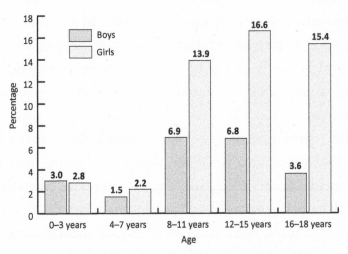

Rates of chronic pain by age groups and gender, as reported in a study by Christel Perquin published in *Pain*.

Women are more likely to have disabling pain—as in, it prevents them from working and fully participating in life—than men. There are some pain conditions in which men outnumber women, such as migraine without aura, cluster headaches and pancreatic disease; however, they are fewer and tend to be rarer than pain conditions affecting women. In a 2007 study on sex and gender differences in pain, researchers listed 38 chronic pain conditions that were more prevalent in women, fifteen more common in men and 24 with no sex difference in prevalence. But the authors didn't list chronic pelvic pain—believed to affect at least 15 per cent of women—which affects all genders as a chronic pain condition. They did, however, list 'pain of psychological origin' as a condition with greater female prevalence. When you start to count chronic pain exclusive to people with female sex organs, such as endometriosis, vulvodynia and vaginismus, the burden of pain conditions is demonstrated to be even greater. In spite of the greater proportion of women than men experiencing pain globally, women's pain is less likely to be treated. This is as true in industrialised nations as it is in developing countries, and is partly down to doctors not believing women's reports of pain and partly due to a lack of effective available treatments.

Even when pain is believed, women's accounts of it are often assumed to be an exaggeration. Once again, we witness the emergence of a form of hysteria—called 'catastrophising' in modern pain-management parlance—when medicine fails to understand the body and can offer no explanation or cure. Pain literature is littered with references to the fact that women catastrophise their pain more than men, and that women are more likely to experience depression and anxiety than men, which are both known triggers for pain. An article on chronic pelvic pain by John Steege and Matthew Siedhoff published in *Obstetrics & Gynecology* defines 'catastrophisation' as: 'the belief that things are as bad as they can be and are not likely to improve'.[9] But it's also known that chronic pain can cause depression and anxiety, that women and others with female sex organs are more susceptible to pain conditions, that they experience more intense pain and pain for longer periods than men, and that their pain is less likely to be treated. Add to this the known lengthy delays in diagnosis of women's chronic pain conditions, and the idea that women are inherently catastrophisers becomes apparent as circular logic.

Women may view their pain as catastrophic to their lives because they haven't been believed by doctors, nurses, family or friends; because they can't get relief from their pain; because they can't go to school, university or work because of their pain; because they witness their career and relationship opportunities dwindle while medicine doesn't ease their pain. And it's important to remember that doctors are trained in a masculinised culture that pathologises women's emotional descriptions of and responses to pain.

Chronic pain is indeed catastrophic for many people. Since we know that mood affects pain perception, noting a tendency to catastrophise is undoubtedly a useful clinical tool if used responsibly. But doctors should also consider medicine's role in women's tendency to catastrophise and be careful in how they treat patients they, or other doctors, have labelled as 'catastrophisers'—good treatment and an understanding doctor could help to reduce catastrophising and improve pain response. In fact, one study on fibromyalgia patients found that those who had more trust in their doctors reported less pain. Based on a survey of 670 people, it also found that those patients who felt medical professionals didn't believe them had a worse quality of life.[10] Pinning pain or symptoms on catastrophisation may do more harm than good.

The Dutch researchers in the children's pain study called for more research into the high prevalence of severe chronic pain and multiple pain in girls aged twelve years and over. That was in 2000, and research since then has started to piece together some of this puzzle. In a 2018 study, the British pain researcher Lydia Coxon wrote:

> Although ongoing pain can reflect continuing tissue damage, pain can also continue beyond normal tissue healing time (approximately 3 months). This 'chronic' pain is not simply a continuation of an acute pain but has its own mechanisms. Although we begin to understand the factors that make an individual at risk of developing chronic pain after an acute injury, the mechanisms maintaining chronic pain and the changes associated with it are remarkably consistent no matter where the pain is perceived or what the underlying pathology is.[11]

It's for this reason, the authors note, that chronic pain must be treated as a disease in its own right and why such a high number of women experience more than one chronic pain condition.

No clear consensus has been reached on why women experience more pain than men, although at least now the question is being studied. What we do know is that this is the case throughout their reproductive lives; in old age, and post-menopause in women, pain tends to even out between everyone, and dementia takes over as the major disease burden for women—another predominantly female condition in which medical science lacks extensive knowledge.

I spoke to one pain researcher who has worked in Australia and the United States to try to understand the gendered differences better. Professor Mark Hutchinson is currently the director of the Australian Research Council Centre of Excellence for Nanoscale BioPhotonics within the University of Adelaide's medical school. From 2005 to 2009, he was working in the world-leading laboratory of Professor Linda Watkins at the Center for Neuroscience at the University of Colorado at Boulder, when the basis for his beliefs about pain differences developed. There, he and Watkins discovered that innate immune receptors in the brain play a role in pain perception and the action of drugs, and that these tend to work differently in male and female brains.

He tells me about the effect this discovery of sex difference had on him as a researcher. 'This was a fascinating area where they—"they", the classic neuroscience community—would say, yes, the male brain is different to the female brain, from neuroanatomical sizes, various processing types with neuronal processors. But the immune part to that really hadn't been explored to any great extent. We invested three-and-a-bit years exploring the immune aspects that may contribute to sex differences in persistent pain processing. What we found was that males and females are fundamentally different in their persistent pain processing.'

What Hutchinson and his fellow researchers discovered was that one type of immune cell, called microglia, has a greater reactivity capacity in females than in males. So the types of immune signals that female microglia send are greater in magnitude and breadth compared to those from male microglia, and this is dependent on a certain female sex hormone. 'We discovered that we could create female-like pain in male rodents just by transferring these microglia from females into males,' Hutchinson says. 'It really had quite a profound impact on me as a pharmacologist because we are developing drugs that are developed in male preclinical rodent models that then go through phase one and phase two clinical trials in males and then to treat a female-predominant pathology. And so that immediately has slight problems.'

This is an understatement: as I pointed out in the introduction, we're currently in a situation where 70 per cent of chronic-pain patients are women but 80 per cent of pain studies are conducted on men or male mice.[12] A 2015 study found that nothing about female persistent pain could be inferred from studying pain in male rodents. It wasn't until 2016 that the US National Institutes of Health made it mandatory for scientists to include female rodents in preclinical pain studies. Other national and international organisations, research institutions and funding organisations are changing their regulations to force scientists to consider sex as a biological variable in all their studies. But we have a lot of catching up to do, and human clinical trials still lag behind in analysing results for sex and gender differences.

In spite of this, Hutchinson envisages a future in which women and men will be prescribed with different treatments to manage chronic pain. 'I think what we need to acknowledge is we're not hitting the right targets in women to treat the persistence of pain because we're using a male-dominated field and we really need to reinvent our toolbox of pharmacological and non-pharmacological treatments to intervene in female persistent pain,' he says.

When I ask him why we're so far behind in what we know about pain compared to other diseases, he says in part it's down to the Western approach to reductionist medicine in which we isolate the body parts and treat them separately. This approach to specialisation is largely based on the seventeenth-century work of René Descartes and often called the Cartesian model of medicine. Hutchinson tells me, 'The problem is that even René Descartes identified that the brain and spinal cord were far too complicated to fit into this model and so he never tried to define the actions of brain and spinal cord. And yet Western medicine has persisted in delineating specialities into systems functions.' So gastroenterologists, cardiologists, renal specialists, urologists and gynaecologists are all working separately on isolated parts and functions of the body. But pain, Hutchinson explains, works across all of these systems and is perceived in the central nervous system. We still don't have the tools to create images of pain in the body; there's not one pain brain centre that researchers can focus on, and how the brain responds to pain is very individualised and depends on many factors, including mood. Pain is an emotional and a sensory integration of a huge amount of information, and it's a response from the brain to another stimulus. 'It's simply far too complicated for our current approaches to research and for medicine to actually imagine and to deal with,' Hutchinson says. 'We are way behind where we should be compared to other disease states.'

Descartes established in Western medicine the strict separation of the body and mind, a concept only now being challenged. He believed pain was a perception of danger, and he described the pain perception pathway as a cord running from the nerve endings to the brain—for example, as your hand goes towards a fire, the heat pulls a cord that rings a bell in the brain. This idea explains acute pain quite well, and helps account for why this pain is fairly well understood and treated, but it's inadequate in explaining chronic pain. Yet for centuries, the origin of pain was believed to be either organic or unexplained. As Maya Dusenbery notes: 'Once this idea—the specificity of pain—took firm hold in American medical schools in the early twentieth century, pain that wasn't explained by an organic pathology came to be seen as hysterical—if the patient's complaint was believed at all.' She adds, quoting medical historian Marcia L. Meldrum, 'Those who suffered from unexplained chronic pain syndromes were often regarded as deluded or were condemned as malingerers or drug abusers.'[13]

Women and others with female reproductive organs who have chronic pain conditions are being told they have medically unexplained symptoms, anxiety, depression or are disbelieved, and have to move from doctor to doctor in order to find a diagnosis or treatment relief. In an exasperating development, 'doctor-shopping' has come to be seen as an indicator that pain is made up, rather than a result of pain that doctors won't believe.

The International Association for the Study of Pain notes: 'Every day millions of women around the world suffer from chronic pain but many remain untreated.'[14] A 2001 paper, 'The girl who cried pain: A bias against women in the treatment of pain',[15] put women's pain on the radar. Not only did the authors, Diane Hoffmann and Anita Tarzian, conclusively show that women experience more pain and for longer periods than men, and are more likely to have chronic pain conditions, but they also presented a smorgasbord of studies proving just how poorly women's pain is treated. These studies show that women were more likely than men to be given sedatives for their pain and vice-versa with narcotics; that both doctors and nurses tended to give women less pain medication after abdominal surgery than men; that post-operatively boys were given more codeine compared to girls and vice-versa with paracetamol; that among both cancer and AIDS patients, women were more likely to be undertreated for their pain than men; that women with chest pain were less likely to be admitted to hospital; and that pain clinics treated women with more minor tranquillisers, antidepressants and non-opioid analgesics than they gave to men, while more opioids were given to men than to women. The authors of one of these studies 'attributed the differences in treatment to the "Yentl Syndrome", i.e., 'women are more likely to be treated less aggressively in their initial encounters with the healthcare system until they "prove that they are as sick as male patients"'.[16]

Hoffmann and Tarzian also documented studies that looked into the reasons for this disparity in treatment. The results throw up predictable contradictions and assumptions, none backed by research. In one study, for example, nurses believed that men felt more pain than women, and that women could cope better with pain than men.[17] Another study 'found that women were frequently thought to be equipped with a "natural capacity to endure pain", in part linked to their reproductive functioning'.[18] But that author, the British academic Gillian Bendelow, rightly pointed out that 'the perceived superiority of capacities of endurance is double-edged for women—the assumption that they may be able to "cope" better may lead to the expectation that they can put up with more pain, that their pain does not need to be taken so seriously'.[19]

Paradoxically, women's better coping strategies for dealing with pain also put them at odds with effective treatment: 'The literature confirms that women in fact have a greater repertoire of coping skills to deal with their pain. These include a greater ability to verbally acknowledge and describe their pain, to seek health-care intervention, and to gain emotional support. Men, in contrast, are likely to ignore the pain or delay seeking treatment.'[20] Yet doctors dismiss women's emotional responses to and descriptions of pain, believing these mean the pain is imaginary or psychogenic.

The International Association for the Study of Pain offers several reasons for why these barriers to treatment still exist: 'Psychosocial factors, such as gender roles, pain coping strategies and mood may influence how pain is perceived and communicated. In addition, there may be a lack of acceptance or understanding of the biological differences between men and women that may impact how pain is perceived. These psychosocial and biological factors, coupled with the economic and political barriers that still exist in many countries, have left millions of women living in pain without proper treatment.'[21]

In 'The girl who cried pain', the authors point to a particular study by New Zealand sociologist Victoria Grace that shows neatly how women's experience of pain is doubted by doctors, and doubly so when medicine lacks knowledge of the underlying condition.[22] '[Grace] found that women with pelvic pain expressed difficulty communicating with their general practitioner about their pain, and some difficulty communicating with their gynecologist. A significant number of the women "did not think the doctor (GP) really understood what they said and left the doctor's office feeling that there were things about their pelvic pain that they hadn't talked about". These women had received 73 different diagnoses to explain the cause of their pain, and reported that their physician implied "nothing was wrong" if no physical cause of pain could be identified. More than half the women said that on occasion they felt that the doctor was not taking their pain seriously or that the doctor expected them to put up with their pain.'

THE PAIN THAT CAN'T BE SEEN

'Pelvic pain in women is one of the last taboos of modern society.'[23] So says the *Pelvic Pain Report*. Chronic pelvic pain is certainly common and has a huge impact on women's lives. One US study found it affected 15 per cent of women, while in the UK the annual prevalence in primary care was 38/1000, a rate similar to that reported for asthma or back pain. A New Zealand study put the figure at 25.4 per cent of women. According to the International Association for the Study of Pain, women complaining of chronic pelvic pain symptoms comprise 15 to 20 per cent of consultations in general gynaecological clinics and up to 10 per cent of all female attendances in general practice. Chronic pelvic pain is the indication for 10 to 15 per cent of hysterectomies performed in the United States.

Women with chronic pelvic pain were found to have undergone almost five times more surgeries and to have sought treatment for four times as many somatic conditions unrelated to their pelvic pain as compared with painfree, agematched controls.[24]

And yet, chronic pelvic pain isn't even mentioned in the British Medical Association's 2018 report, *Addressing Unmet Needs in Women's Health*, or in the Australian government's National Women's Health Policy of 2010 . . . except in a brief one-sentence mention of pelvic pain as a possible consequence of pelvic inflammatory disease as a result of chlamydia. Neither of these documents addresses the lifelong impact of chronic pain conditions on women. There's something deeply disturbing about the acceptance of women's suffering exemplified in these documents' complete ignorance of pain as a major factor in women's lives. As the journalist Caroline Reilly wrote in her heartbreaking 2018 essay for Rewire News, 'Every woman I know is in pain.'[25] In *Fleabag*, Kristin Scott Thomas's character Belinda delivers a powerful speech about women's pain: 'Women are born with pain built in. It's our physical destiny: period pains, sore boobs, you know. We carry it within ourselves throughout our lives, men don't.'[26]

The *Pelvic Pain Report* noted the effect this ignorance has on women's lives: 'Its stigma permeates every aspect of her care from her parents' perception of their daughter's complaints, through the lack of integrated health services to the absence of pelvic pain as a worthwhile subject for clinical research.'[27]

The article on this topic by Steege and Siedhoff called for greater understanding of chronic pelvic pain and its official recognition as a disease state in itself. The paper defined chronic pelvic pain as 'noncyclic pain of 6 or more months' duration that localizes to the anatomic pelvis, anterior abdominal wall at or below the umbilicus, the lumbosacral back or the buttocks, and is of sufficient severity to cause functional disability or lead to medical care'.[28] The paper estimated the cost to the US economy to be in excess of US$3 billion; the Australian *Pelvic Pain Report* put the figure for the cost to the Australian economy at A$6.6 billion,[29] acknowledging this was likely to be conservative since it was based on what was known about endometriosis—just one of several pelvic pain conditions—and didn't include indirect costs.

Even reports focusing on the impact of chronic diseases fail to mention chronic pelvic pain—or even endometriosis, about which more is known. Chronic pelvic pain affects the same number of women as diabetes and more women than asthma, two chronic diseases that receive a great deal of attention and research money because they also affect a lot of men— though often the impacts of chronic pelvic pain, which men also get although at lower numbers than women, are more severe in terms of economic cost and quality of life than these other diseases. Other chronic pain conditions such as fibromyalgia, painful bladder syndrome, irritable bowel syndrome and chronic fatigue syndrome are rarely mentioned in such documents.

As with all pain conditions, chronic pelvic pain in the past was believed to purely represent physical, visible disease within the pelvis. Where endometriosis, ovarian cysts or adhesions were found, this was thought to fully explain the pain, and where no such pathology could be found the pain was a mystery, unexplained or psychosomatic. 'Traditional thinking about chronic pelvic pain has emphasized observable organic pathology (e.g., endometriosis, adhesions), but the connection between these problems and pain symptoms is actually more tenuous than previously thought,' Steege and Siedhoff wrote in their paper on chronic pelvic pain. They added: 'More and more data confirming the coexistence of one or more other chronic pain disorders in patients—conditions such as interstitial cystitis (also known as painful bladder syndrome), irritable bowel syndrome, temporomandibular joint disorder, migraine headaches, vulvodynia, and fibromyalgia—suggest that perhaps we should be treating pelvic pain itself as the disease rather than as just a manifestation of a specific pathologic change.'[30]

An Australian researcher from the University of Sydney, Alison Hey-Cunningham, has found women who have endometriosis are 180 times more likely to also report chronic fatigue syndrome than the general female population.[31] The International Association for the Study of Pain notes that about 20 per cent of people with endo also have other chronic pain conditions such as irritable bowel syndrome, interstitial cystitis/painful bladder syndrome, vulvodynia, temporomandibular joint disorder, migraine or fibromyalgia, and/or autoimmune disorders such as systemic lupus erythematosus, rheumatoid arthritis, chronic fatigue syndrome and Sjögren's syndrome.[32] There is obviously more to pelvic pain than just what is seen within the pelvis.

In the 2018 HBO drama *Sharp Objects*, Jackie, played by Elizabeth Perkins, shows Camille, played by Amy Adams, a trinket box full of pills. 'I got endometriosis, pelvic floor dysfunction, I got cysts, IC, IBS, and fibromyalgia,' she says as she pulls a new pill out for each diagnosis. Then she adds: 'Oh, and hypochondria! I've been diagnosed, and undiagnosed, re-diagnosed, all that.'[33] But calling herself a hypochondriac belies the fact that her particular collection of conditions is not at all uncommon. I have endometriosis, pelvic floor muscle problems and endometriomas, which are cysts in my ovaries, and at one point, it was suggested I might have IBS.

But there's a growing recognition that the pain symptoms reported are not at all random. Ten chronic pain conditions in particular cluster together in women to paint a common pain picture. These are endometriosis (often associated with painful periods), vulvodynia, temporomandibular disorders, chronic fatigue syndrome, irritable bowel syndrome, painful bladder syndrome (also called IC, interstitial cystitis), fibro-myalgia, chronic tension-type headache, migraine headache, and chronic low back pain. They often also have pelvic muscle dysfunction and spasm. The US Congress and National Insti-tutes of Health have described the clustering of these conditions as Chronic Overlapping Pain Conditions (COPCs) in order to recognise their relation to each other. They recognise that not all women with pain have all these conditions but having one of them increases the chance they will have or develop other pain conditions within this group. The Chronic Pain Research Alliance, an NGO advocating for better understand-ing of chronic overlapping pain conditions, says that more than 50 million Americans may be affected by COCPs at a cost of at least US$80 billion annually in direct and indirect healthcare expenses. Unfortunately, the billions of dollars spent don't always buy sufferers lasting relief. While some women do well with current treatments, others undergo repeated medical visits and multiple invasive interventions without relief.

Many women with these conditions are 'diagnosed, undiagnosed, and re-diagnosed'. Pelvic pain in women is due for a major review: a new start looking at how and why it happens.

Pain researchers believe that a process called central sensitisation plays a major part in chronic pain conditions. The website Pain Science explains central sensitisation:

> Pain itself often modifies the way the central nervous system works, so that a patient actually becomes more sensitive and gets *more pain* with *less provocation*. It's called 'central sensitization' because it involves changes in the *central* nervous system (CNS) in particular—the brain and the spinal cord. Sensitized patients are not only more sensitive to things that should hurt, but sometimes to ordinary touch and pressure as well. Their pain also 'echoes', fading more slowly than in other people.[34]

So the source of the pain is not just in the pelvis but in the spinal cord and brain as well. This provides at least part of the explanation for the wide range of symptoms, and why pain can continue after removal of the primary source of the problem, such as pain that persists after surgical removal of endometriosis lesions or the uterus itself.

I'm focusing on chronic pelvic pain because that's my experience and because I have access to Dr Susan Evans, a pelvic pain expert, to explain it.

In Evans' inner-city Adelaide home, her large office is well-equipped for pelvic pain patients and I'm offered a variety of chairs: the soft low sofa is comfy but often not suitable for people with pelvic pain; there are higher chairs and orthopaedic chairs and office chairs. I opt for the low sofa because I've taken a variety of painkillers and believe I can handle the terrible pain I awoke with. I try to disguise my difficulty getting in and out of the chair even though I'm here to speak to a world expert on this kind of pain, while writing a book with the aim of making it easier to talk about this kind of pain. I want to be here as a journalist, not a patient.

Not only is Evans sharp, articulate and passionate, she is also caring and inquisitive, and after some earl grey tea and Florentines, I end up—perhaps inappropriately—divulging my entire medical history over the course of our two mornings spent together. Evans is the first person to make sense of all my symptoms while helping me fully appreciate these notions of central sensitisation that I've been grappling with.

Primarily interested in pelvic pain, Evans echoes the sentiments of Steege and Siedhoff in thinking that chronic pelvic pain is a disease state in itself. She co-founded the Pelvic Pain Foundation of Australia in 2015 after writing a book on endo and pelvic pain in 2005 in order to improve the lives of people with these conditions, 'because I had been thinking for quite a while that women with pain were getting lost in the health system and that really they needed a bit of help on understanding what was good treatment and what wasn't good treatment'. Evans is a gynaecologist and specialist pain physician who is writing her PhD on dysmenorrhea in order to further understand chronic pelvic pain and the role of period pain as a trigger for later chronic pain states. She works closely with Mark Hutchinson, and they've both come to believe that the innate immune system and its role in inflammation is the key to unlocking what's happening in chronic pain conditions.

This takes me back to Angela Saini's book *Inferior* and the role of the female immune system in our longer lives and greater prevalence for autoimmune conditions.

When we get to the point in Evans' explanation of how chronic pelvic pain works, we move from the sofa to her multifunctional desk, where she moves from showing me papers and slides on computer screens to drawing diagrams on paper. I am enthralled. Her current obsession is with gender and pain; she calls it the next frontier in medicine and is devoted to drawing attention to the issues and to finding greater understanding herself. She shows me the Dutch study on pain in children. 'You can see the gender pain disadvantage starting once girls get near puberty. They start to outpace the boys when it comes to pain. They did nothing wrong, they only grew up. By the time girls reach sixteen to eighteen years, they are three to four times as likely as boys to have a persistent pain condition. And the girls have more days of pain, and more pain symptoms, despite the boys doing higher risk activities. The whole thing is totally not fair but that's what happens to girls.'

Evans continues: 'Throughout life, almost all pain conditions are more common in women than men.' In addition to pelvic pain and migraine, Evans points to irritable bowel syndrome, fibromyalgia and rheumatoid arthritis as pain conditions that affect women more often than men. I point out that many of them are contested: not believed by doctors. She puts this down to the fact that these are 'pains that can't be seen'. Unlike the acute pain of a broken bone with obvious changes on an X-ray, there may be nothing to see on scans or in an operation in people with chronic pain.

'Humans have always struggled to understand pain that can't be seen. It's too easy for others to imagine it isn't real,' she tells me. This is exacerbated in conditions that relate to pelvic pain—what can be seen at an operation may just be part of the pain picture. It doesn't always describe the full extent of the suffering or symptoms. It's also beset by stigmas and taboos that make it difficult for women to talk about their sex organs or anything related to them.

Evans begins drawing on a diagram of the female reproductive organs as she explains how pelvic pain works. She draws into the diagram the pelvic floor muscles and obturator internus—muscles that often lead to the most severe pain in chronic pelvic pain patients: the stabbing or aching pains. In pelvic pain, unsurprisingly, the pain usually starts in the pelvis, often with period pain. That pain sends a signal up the spinal cord into the brain, but it also sends messages to surrounding muscles, telling them to tighten up. Endo lesions, which become inflamed, also send signals up the spinal cord into the brain and to pelvic muscles. These constant signals to and from the brain end up sensitising the nerve pathways.

In pelvic pain patients, the uterus may be the first organ to cause pain, but soon the bladder and bowel start to send pain signals too. Over time, pelvic pain patients often develop sensitivity in the bowel or bladder and may be diagnosed with irritable bowel syndrome, food intolerances, painful bladder syndrome/interstitial cystitis, and—sometimes incorrectly— urinary tract infections. This isn't usually a structural problem with the bowel or bladder (although sometimes endo can attach or form lesions to these organs), but an increase in sensitivity of the organs. They react more to specific foods (bowel)

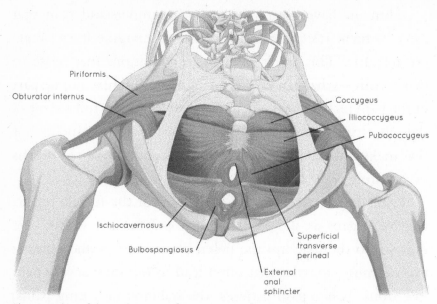

The muscles of the pelvis are often sources of severe pain
Source: Illustration by Pelvic Guru in partnership with the Global Pelvic Health Alliance, www.pelvicguru.com

or normal filling (bladder) than they used to. 'Viscero-visceral hyperalgesia' is the term used to describe the idea that 'when one organ's unhappy, they're all unhappy', Evans says. There's also a problem with the way the brain controls pain. Communication between the pelvis and the brain goes both ways. As well as pain signals heading up the spinal cord to the brain to inform it of possible danger, lovely calming signals called descending inhibition send messages to the pelvis telling it not to worry about sensations it knows are OK. This stops us from feeling functions that we don't need to feel—like our bladder starting to fill, or our bowel functioning normally. We don't need to feel what's in the bladder until it's time to empty it, and same goes with the bowel—there's no good reason for us to notice every step of the digestive process. Equally, we don't need to feel which muscles are being used to keep us sitting on a chair, or the feeling of clothes against our skin. The descending inhibitory messages are the good ones. Trouble is, people with chronic pain seem to lose these. They start to notice sensations more. Normal sensations become painful, painful sensations become more painful, and sometimes there can be pain when nothing at all is happening. And this is what happens in chronic pelvic pain.

Over time, pelvic muscles become tighter and tighter, and may be sore to the touch. The muscles can ache or spasm, causing stabbing pains in the abdomen, sides, up the vagina and/or rectum, or can be felt as pain down the front of the legs and into the back. This pain can also lead to vaginismus or vulvodynia. It's what Evans calls the 'worst pain'. 'And of course it's a pain that can't be seen: blood tests, scans, laparoscopies, can be totally normal,' she says. (I now have a Post-it note stuck to my computer that reads: 'UNTENSE'. Whenever I see it, I remember to relax the muscles of my glutes, inner thighs and pelvic floor—this isn't easy but I'm practising!)

Three key factors are important here. One, pain usually starts in the pelvis, often with endo lesions or period pain. Two, muscles tighten and cause aches and pains in the back, legs, hips, vagina and/or vulva. Three, the inflammatory response of the innate immune system releases small proteins called cytokines to induce what Evans calls the 'feel bad' symptoms of anxiety, low mood, fatigue, poor sleep, nausea, dizziness and feeling faint. Cytokines are involved in lots of functions and, Evans explains, are what make you feel bad when you have the flu, for example.

To Evans and Hutchinson, inflammation is the key factor

in all of this—they believe that endometriosis, pelvic pain and possibly fertility issues as well are all potential consequences of that inflammation. Evans says: 'What people often think, which I think is all wrong, is that you get the endo, then you get the pelvic pain. In other words, the endo probably acting via inflammation causes the pain. There's loads of evidence that the endo doesn't fit with the amount of pain. So the way I see it is that this underlying thing we call inflammation, which is poorly understood, can show up in different ways. It can increase the chance of endo lesions. It can cause pain. And it can result—in some people—in fertility issues.' This theory would explain a lot.

Currently most doctors believe that endo is caused by retrograde menstruation, which is when menstrual blood flows from the uterus into the pelvic cavity instead of being expelled from the body through the vagina. Except most women experience retrograde menstruation but only 10 per cent have endo—a fact that is left unexplained by the retrograde theory. What Evans is saying is that most women's immune systems get rid of that excess blood; in women with endo, the immune system *doesn't* get rid of the blood and lesions form. So the question that now needs answering is this: what is happening to these women's immune systems that prevents them from expelling the stray blood?

We know that endo isn't the only cause of chronic pelvic pain: while 82 per cent of women with chronic pelvic pain have endo, it's well known that some endo sufferers don't experience associated pelvic pain at all.[35] To put it simply: not all women with chronic pelvic pain have endometriosis and not all women with endometriosis have chronic pelvic pain.

'This model just doesn't explain the full range of symptoms women experience,' Evans says.

British researchers Katy Vincent, Lydia Coxon and Andrew Horne have also shown that 'these central changes are not due to endometriosis itself, but rather the pain that arises from it. The same group have carried out many studies in patients with fibromyalgia with similar (although subtly different) findings, further highlighting the similarities between endometriosis-associated pain and other chronic pain conditions.'[36]

Hutchinson's research, Evans explains to me, leads them to believe that aspects of the immune system called toll-like receptors, which act on glial cells in the nervous system, are active in modifying pain impulses. It's early days for these ideas, Evans is careful to point out, and we have a way to go yet, but it's a theory she believes helps explain a lot of what is going on in chronic pelvic pain and is informing future research projects. She fleshes out the theory for me with another diagram: 'The process we now loosely call "inflammation" acts via special receptors on cells called toll-like receptors to sensitise the body to pain.' What's causing the inflammation, and how we can stop that happening, is where focused research could have potentially great results for a multitude of chronic pain conditions.

It's hard not to get excited by Evans' zeal. I know she's describing pain, lost opportunities and intense sadness for many women, but it feels like a huge breakthrough in understanding conditions she's been treating for 20 years. 'Now the really interesting thing,' she tells me, 'is this describes what a woman comes with, this describes all of her symptoms generally.'

As discussed in the last chapter, Evans' 2018 study showed

that women with dysmenorrhea (with or without endo-metriosis) had an average of eight-and-a-half other symptoms from a possible fourteen, including stabbing pains in the pelvis, bowel problems (often diagnosed as IBS), food intolerances, bladder problems, headaches, sexual pain, vulval pain, fatigue, poor sleep, nausea, sweating, dizziness/faint, anxiety and low mood. Less than 1 per cent of the women in the study experienced period pain alone without any other symptoms.[37] These are the symptoms that women and other people with female sex organs come complaining of to Evans.

Until now, medical science has not been able to account for the wide variety of symptoms or how they were associated. Evans breaks down what we now know about the chronic pain condition: it's worse with poor sleep, stress, oestrogens and opioids. It's better with regular exercise that isn't too intense, pain psychology and a drug called amitriptyline, which acts on the central nervous system. Amitriptyline (the Australian brand name is Endep) is what's called a tricyclic antidepressant. It's a drug that was once used to treat anxiety and depression but today is mostly used in low doses to treat chronic pain. It's readily available in most Western countries by prescription from a medical practitioner and while it can make you sleepy, has relatively few side effects in the low doses taken to treat chronic pain. Evans adds, cautiously, that maybe testosterone could also help with chronic pain—but she draws a big question mark over that and I'll come back to it shortly. There's also some evidence that curcumin, found in turmeric, can be helpful— but it's difficult to eat enough of it in a normal diet to make a difference to pain.

So what's activating the immune system? Here we get into

loads of theories. Some researchers have proposed that a history of trauma—sexual abuse is commonly suggested—could be a cause. However, not all people with chronic pain conditions, or chronic pelvic pain specifically, have been sexually abused, so this theory doesn't stack up. Evans' 2018 study found that less than 20 per cent of pelvic pain patients studied had experienced a distressing sexual event in their past, although those who did reported a significantly higher number of symptoms and pain on more days than women without this history.[38] Steege and Siedhoff included this cautionary note in their study of chronic pelvic pain:

> In relation to pain, abuse, particularly that which occurs in formative years, may serve to alter the response to nociception and central pain processing. That said, not all abused patients go on to have chronic pain nor do all patients with pain have a history of abuse, so it might be the response to trauma that plays a key role in development of chronic pain. Health care providers need to take into account the presence of abuse in a patient's history when detected but be careful to avoid necessarily concluding a causal relationship in that patient's pain.[39]

Another theory suggests that exposure to a virus, bacteria or toxins may also kick off this immune response. A group of Japanese researchers have recently proposed the bacterial contamination hypothesis as an explanation. Their study, published in *Reproductive Medicine and Biology* in 2018, found higher rates of *E. coli* bacteria in the menstrual blood of women with endometriosis compared to those who didn't have endo, and that this kicked off an inflammatory response in the innate immune system via the toll-like receptors.[40]

A third theory suggests that period pain itself could be the trigger that leads to pain sensitisation and the development of chronic pain conditions. Katy Vincent, whose work I've mentioned before, is a consultant gynaecologist and senior pain fellow at the Nuffield Department of Women's & Reproductive Health at Oxford University. She has a special interest in female pain and the role of the central nervous system in generating and maintaining pain in women. She's also interested in how pain interacts with steroid hormones: those such as oestrogen, progesterone and testosterone produced in the ovaries and testes, as well as hormones produced in the adrenal glands. In 2011 Vincent published an influential study, 'Dysmenorrhoea is associated with central changes in otherwise healthy women', showing that period pain could lead to central pain sensitisation.[41] The study focused on women who had period pain but didn't have chronic pelvic pain or report pain outside menstruation. In other words, apart from the period pain, they considered themselves well. But the study found they were more susceptible to pain throughout their cycle and were sensitised in parts of their body other than their abdomens. Vincent concluded that the experience of having period pain made a woman more sensitive to pain throughout her cycle.

While Vincent has acknowledged it's hard to know without further study whether the alterations in the central nervous system and hypothalamic–pituitary–ovarian axis are a cause or effect of repeated episodes of pain, they do point to the possibility that period pain could predispose women to developing chronic pain conditions after a minor incident. The example she gives is the development of irritable bowel syndrome after a bout of gastroenteritis. She writes that period pain could also 'partly contribute to the gender differences observed in the prevalence of chronic pain conditions'.[42]

Evans, a close follower of Vincent's work, conducted a follow-up clinical study in Australia, with Gemma Hardi and Meredith Craigie, to show that untreated period pain could lead to later chronic pain conditions. Their study demonstrates that period pain can progress to chronic pelvic pain—as quickly as one year, or as late as 30 years after severe period pain started. Girls even as young as eleven could be affected. 'Adolescent populations may be at particular risk of central changes and transition to chronic pain due to the greater plasticity of their nervous systems,' the authors wrote.[43] This has huge implications, not only for medicine but for society as well. The messages that period pain is normal and the afflicted should suffer in silence are potentially setting women up for a lifetime of pain.

This is a major factor in the long delays women face in diagnosis. They delay going to the doctor to treat pain conditions for a number of reasons: they're busy with work, home life, relationships and caring responsibilities; they're taught to believe that period pain is normal; they live in a society where women are expected to endure suffering without complaint; they think they won't be believed; they think their pain is normal; they've been socialised to gain self-worth through pleasing others, so focusing on their own health may be viewed as selfish, particularly when they're caring for other ill family members.

In 'The girl who cried pain', Hoffman and Tarzian concluded that women's pain is undertreated for numerous reasons: 'the literature supports the conclusion that there are gender-based biases regarding women's pain experiences. These biases have led healthcare providers to discount women's self-reports of pain at least until there is objective evidence for the pain's cause. Medicine's focus on objective factors and its cultural stereotypes of women combine insidiously, leaving women at greater risk for inadequate pain relief and continued suffering.'[44]

This is why education in schools in so important. New Zealand already has a schools program, known as the ME— Menstrual Education program—that addresses period pain. After participating in it, 29 per cent of girls have said they're aware that their menstrual symptoms and pain may not be normal, and this has led to increased trends in presentation of symptoms to doctors, intervention and early diagnosis.[45] Evans is one of those behind a similar program—developed by the Pelvic Pain Foundation, called Periods, Pain and Endometriosis (PPEP-Talk Program)—being trialled in South Australia. It's urgent that pain is included in any lessons about menstruation so that all students understand it better.

Doctors must also be educated to treat period pain more seriously—and given we know women delay seeking attention, doctors should respond quickly to these complaints. An influential study by Melissa Parker on Australian girls found that 93 per cent of them experience some period pain. About 20 per cent experience severe pain, 24 per cent say their period interferes with four out of nine life activities, and 26 per cent miss school because of pain.[46] So a quarter of girls are missing school because of pain, and nobody thinks it's a problem?

What opportunities are lost for girls who miss days of school each month because of period pain? What sports have these girls stopped participating in because of pain? What school work has been missed? What friendships have been lost? What has happened to these girls' self-esteem?

The good news is that although it has taken millennia, it seems that now, finally, medicine is beginning to acknowledge the severity of some women's period pain. In 2016 John Guillebaud, a professor of reproductive health at University College London, made international headlines when he said that period pain could be 'almost as bad as having a heart attack', telling *Quartz* magazine: 'Men don't get it and it hasn't been given the centrality it should have. I do believe it's something that should be taken care of, like anything else in medicine.'[47]

But it's clear that further study is needed into the experience of menstrual pain. What little research we have has focused on biological sex differences, whereas it's clear that gender plays a role in pain, and how treatment is delivered and sought, so it should be a focus in the future. Gender is a fluid idea that varies across cultures and changes over time, and so it's much harder to study than biological sex—but difficulty shouldn't prevent progress. One key study of the effect of hormones in pain was undertaken in transgender men and women over the process of transition. Those who transitioned to women developed more pain conditions after transition and an increase in pain severity of pain conditions present before transition. Those who transitioned to men reported a decrease in pain after they transitioned.[48] Those hormones certainly seem to have a role.

There's a developing theory in pain research that testosterone protects men against pain. Until recently, most of the research into female pain focused on oestrogen as a sensitiser, but researchers are starting to believe that while this may play a part, it's not the full story—they believe that testosterone may play a larger role in protecting men from pain than previously understood. Some of Katy Vincent's research has shown that women on the combined oral contraceptive pill with lower testosterone levels experienced more pain than those who had higher testosterone levels. A 2015 study showed an improvement in fibromyalgia symptoms after testosterone treatment in women with low testosterone levels.[49] Testosterone treatment in women remains a controversial issue, and while this research is in its infancy, this is a debate well worth having. Another recent development in pain research suggests that sex differences in pain may be produced directly by sex chromosome (X and Y) genes, rather than by gonadal hormones.[50]

Chronic pain is a severe burden on women. Even those in Vincent's study who had period pain but were otherwise well reported lower quality-of-life scores than those who didn't have period pain. As we've seen, chronic pain can have a negative effect on education, careers, relationships, social activities and fertility. In Australia, endometriosis alone causes afflicted women to lose eleven working hours per week in absenteeism (absence from work due to pain) and presenteeism (working less effectively due to pain), according to the *Pelvic Pain Report*. In Ireland, the US, the UK and Italy, the average extra cost per week to the employer is $200 to $250/week in absenteeism and presenteeism.[51] Women's opportunities are being severely limited by pain—this has a cost to the sufferers themselves, their families, friends and loved ones, and also to society as a whole.

We have to stop believing that pain is a natural state for women.

When I had a broken back, I couldn't move and couldn't speak, and my movement was limited. When I had a broken shoulder, combined with all the sprains, bruising and lacerations from the train accident, I was similarly limited. This is what doctors look for when they ask about pain. A compound fracture of the sacrum is a ten, and no one even needs to ask: they can see a ten, they know what it looks like. You can't be texting your friends or looking at Facebook when you're in ten out of ten pain.

But chronic pain is different. It doesn't fit the acute pain scale—a fact now widely acknowledged in the pain medicine field.

On my worst pain days with endometriosis and adenomyosis, I'm still huddled over, grasping my abdomen, hobbling with hip pain, or rubbing the front of my right leg or interrupted suddenly by sharp stabbing pains to my abdomen. Some days the pain and nausea combined are so bad, I can't move. Is this pain a ten? No, but I feel so much worse than I did while lying in bed with a dose of morphine recovering from a fracture. I feel *bad*. I feel fatigued, which isn't the same thing as feeling tired. I've felt tired too—I had insomnia in my 20s and early 30s, and it was hell. But the intense fatigue that overcomes me with pelvic pain isn't like that—it's like walking through sludge wearing a suit of armour. Yes, I can go to work, probably even do what needs to be done. But it's so hard; my brain is foggy. Thinking feels like driving a car with a dirty windscreen while wearing smudged glasses.

More than anything, more than having a baby, I want this pain and fatigue fixed.

CHAPTER 7

Time to ditch the bikini: the women's health conditions you never hear about

When we think of women's health, what comes to mind? Most people probably think of the female reproductive system. Pregnancy, giving birth, abortion, menstruation, menopause and breast cancer—that's what women's health is, isn't it? That's certainly how medicine has treated it. Maternal and reproductive health are undoubtedly a major part of women's health and deserve the widespread attention they receive. However, it's particularly cruel to witness the advancements made in these areas stop at class, race, ethnic and national borders. The risk of a woman in a developing country dying from a maternal-related cause is about 33 times higher than that of a woman in a developed nation, according to the World Health Organization, which says, 'maternal mortality is a health indicator that shows very wide gaps between rich and poor, urban and rural areas, both between countries and within them'.[1] There are also broad disparities in race witnessed within countries.

In April 2018, the *New York Times Magazine* published an article by Linda Villarosa that sent shockwaves around the world. Titled 'Why America's black mothers and babies are in a life-or-death crisis', this article plagued my mind for months on end. Villarosa has documented a body of research gathered over the past few decades that shows the experience of being a black woman in America is so stressful, it has led to increasingly high rates of death and illness in black mothers and their children, regardless of their class or education. In fact, babies born to college-educated black parents were twice as likely to die as those born to similarly educated white parents.

'The United States is one of only thirteen countries in the world where the rate of maternal mortality—the death of a woman related to pregnancy or childbirth up to a year after the end of pregnancy—is now worse than it was 25 years ago,' Villarosa notes.[2] Black women are three to four times as likely to die from pregnancy-related causes as white women in America; black infants are more than twice as likely to die as white infants. According to Villarosa:

> For black women in America, an inescapable atmosphere of societal and systemic racism can create a kind of toxic physiological stress, resulting in conditions—including hypertension and pre-eclampsia—that lead directly to higher

rates of infant and maternal death. And that societal racism is further expressed in a pervasive, long-standing racial bias in health care—including the dismissal of legitimate concerns and symptoms—that can help explain poor birth outcomes even in the case of black women with the most advantages.[3]

I couldn't stop thinking about this article. It demonstrates the need for intersectional feminism by revealing how the combination of racism and sexism is more than the sum of its parts: it's deadly.

I couldn't begin to imagine the anguish of black women reading that story or experiencing that treatment, but I wondered if Aboriginal and Torres Strait Islander women were having similar experiences in Australia. When I ask Aboriginal women, their answer is, 'Almost certainly.'

One of them is Janine Mohamed, the CEO of the Congress of Aboriginal and Torres Strait Islander Nurses and Midwives. She spends a lot of time explaining to doctors and to the public how racism affects health, and has spent her career advocating for, and delivering, better healthcare services to Aboriginal and Torres Strait Islander people.

While the maternal and infant mortality rates for Indigenous Australians aren't as bad as for black people in America, they're still disgraceful, especially in a country that prides itself on its universal healthcare system—and ten years after a national program was launched to close the gap between the health, education and life outcomes of Indigenous and non-Indigenous Australians. From 2012 to 2014, Indigenous women were almost two and a half times more likely to die in childbirth than non-Indigenous women.[4]

Mohamed has been instrumental in developing Birthing-on-Country programs in Aboriginal communities, which include high quality, culturally sensitive prenatal and postnatal care in conjunction with Aboriginal community-controlled health services. These programs have seen improvements in maternal health and mortality, as well as improvements in infant health and mortality.[5] But when I ask her what she thinks the most urgent health priority is for Aboriginal and Torres Strait Islander women, her answer is clear: 'culturally safe and respectful services'. Of course maternal and child mortality and morbidity are important to her, as are cardio-vascular disease and diabetes, which disproportionately affect Aboriginal and Torres Strait Islander people. (They're also overrepresented in polycystic ovary syndrome and some auto-immune conditions.) But no single disease can be a priority until Aboriginal people can feel safe walking into a hospital, or can access good-quality healthcare where they live. Health-care services, she tells me, have been developed for where most people live, not for those most in need.

A failure of Indigenous women to access prenatal care is often given as a major factor in the difference in maternal and infant mortality and morbidity figures between Indigenous and non-Indigenous people in official reports. But Mohamed points out that the biggest factor involved in whether an Indig-enous person will access health services is their prior experience of that service: 'A lot of non-Aboriginal people working in policy will think that we don't go to services because we're not interested in our health. But in actual fact, the biggest determinant is actually our experiences with health services—and what we see happening.'

After reporting on the Naomi Williams inquest, I had the opportunity to speak to a nurse who worked in the town Williams was from. She told me she'd recently seen an Aboriginal woman who'd begged not to be sent to the local hospital when she was referred there. The nurse recalled the look of fear on the patient's face and worried how many other Aboriginal people in the small country town might be refusing to seek help for their health because of the fear of the hospital induced by Williams' death.

A hospital should be a place of safety for everyone. This doesn't seem like much to ask in one of the world's richest countries, and one with a supposedly universal healthcare system. But some problems related to ill health in women and other minority people can't be fixed by the healthcare system alone—throughout this book, we've seen how social factors contribute to the development of chronic physical and mental health issues. But it would make a good start to have a health-care system with the default of believing what all patients report, alongside a research community that considers the full picture of everyone's health and ceases to think of the male body as the default human being.

I tell these stories in order to emphasise that even where we've made great strides—'almost nothing else in medicine has saved lives on the scale that obstetrics has,' wrote the American surgeon and public health researcher Atul Gawande in a 2006 *New Yorker* article[6]—these gains haven't been spread evenly among populations, even populations living as neigh-bours. It should remain a priority for medicine, governments and society to close these gaps in infant and maternal health.

But I also want to point out that the focus on reproduc-tion as the beginning and end of women's health and the cheerleading over their longer life span have obscured the true picture of women's lives. Dr Nanette Wenger drew attention to this in calling medicine's focus on women's health a 'bikini approach' with the rest of the woman ignored.[7] It's the very reason the US Office of Research on Women's Health was established in the 1990s.

In this book, I've tried to fill in the gaps in women's health that aren't often talked about. I don't think women are living as well as we should be. As we have already seen, we're more likely to suffer severe disability than men of the same age and more likely to have multiple chronic illnesses, and although we live longer than men, we live fewer active years. The *Relieving Pain in America* report outlined a number of studies that have shown a link between chronic pain and suicide. A Canadian population-based study found the presence of one or more chronic pain conditions is associated with suicide ideation and suicide attempts, even after adjusting for mental disorders.[8] Gender is a key determinant of health. Racism, poverty, violence, trauma, abuse and stress all contribute to poor health, and women suffer disproportionately in many of these areas. I think this has largely been ignored in Western approaches to women's health.

According to the Chronic Pain Research Alliance, the ten chronic overlapping pain conditions are particularly poorly understood and plagued by stigma, delayed diagnosis, a lack of coordinated care, and poor evidence on safe and effective treatments. People with chronic pain illnesses and auto-immune conditions face lengthy delays in diagnosis, along with disbelief and piecemeal care. Sufferers who are women of colour, LGBTI+ people and other minority women face tougher battles to be heard, believed and treated.

While depression and anxiety are widely understood to be linked to chronic pain and autoimmune conditions, they aren't always treated together. And government policies on mental health rarely address chronic pain and autoimmune conditions as contributory factors to mental illness. We know that people who have these conditions have a better quality of life when they have a trusting relationship with their doctor. We know chronic pain can lead to depression and depression can make chronic pain worse.

After four years of listening to women with these conditions, I'd wager a bet that good medical care, being listened to, believed and receiving treatment that eases pain and fatigue would go a long way to reducing the depression and anxiety that accompanies many of these conditions. Certainly from my own experience, I'm infinitely happier when I'm not racked with pain or fatigue. I'm lucky to have a GP and a gynaecologist who listen to my priorities and believe my reports of my own health. It's not rocket science—because there *are* treatments that work. For me, a combination of surgery, pelvic physiotherapy, amitriptyline and hormonal birth control have worked well and I now have a generally good quality of life. There are many others like me. They may not respond to the same combination of treatments but they do find good doctors and satisfactory therapies and happily go about their lives.

But there remains, in all aspects of healthcare delivery, a received impression that difficult women get chronic pain. That somehow, women who have complex pain conditions have an attitude problem or that the sole cause of their pain is an experience of trauma that's out of the hands of most doctors to treat; that they're attention seekers, they can't face life, they don't *want* to be well. Doctors—and nurses—everywhere look for a secondary gain these women might have in being sick, in pain, depressed. And there's a suggestion that if only they could be a little more positive, everything would be OK.

That's hysteria, right there, persisting among us.

This is not to say that everyone with complex problems and generalised pain *will* have a chronic pain or autoimmune condition. But it shouldn't be the default assumption that women with symptoms of generalised pain, distress and fatigue are all somatisers or simply anxious about their health. The lengthy delays in diagnosis common across the world in debilitating conditions that solely or predominantly affect women show far too many doctors still hold this default view. Shouldn't the onus be on the doctor to investigate first and diagnose later?

The *Relieving Pain in America* report claimed that 'effective pain management is a moral imperative'. To date, Western healthcare systems have failed women in that moral imperative.

Celebrities are perhaps doing more today to build a full picture of women's health than medicine. Lena Dunham has drawn a huge amount of much-needed attention to endometriosis. She also suffers from fibromyalgia and the mixed connective tissues disorder, Ehlers–Danlos syndrome. In an Instagram post in 2018, Dunham described the pain from fibromyalgia: 'My ankles and wrists were weak and my fingers didn't do their assigned job. Yesterday I felt like I was suspended in gel, and when I meditated a line of pain zipped from my neck to my foot.' She also stated: 'This is fibromyalgia. It's little understood and so even though I have a lot of knowledge and support it's hard to shake the feeling that I am crazy.'[9]

Lady Gaga has been vocal about her struggle with

fibromyalgia. In her 2017 documentary, *Gaga: Five Foot Two*, she shows viewers, in excruciating detail, how her chronic pain interrupts her life and causes her great anguish. In one scene, she describes her pain to a doctor like this: 'It's tension in my abdomen and it just feels like my muscles are gripping all around my intestines and it's so inflamed. And my hip hurts every single day.' In another scene, she is lying on a sofa, crying. 'The whole right side of my body is in a . . . I don't know, spasm. It feels like there's a rope from my first toe all the way up my leg and around my first rib and to my shoulder, then my neck and head, jaw. My fucking face hurts.' She also recognises her privilege in being able to have her pain treated by multiple health professionals—a luxury so many people with chronic pain simply can't afford. She says, 'I just think of all the other people who have maybe something like this that are struggling to figure out what it is and they don't have the money to have somebody help them. I don't know what I'd do.'[10] In a 2018 interview with *Vogue*, she said, 'I get so irritated with people who don't believe fibromyalgia is real . . . People need to be more compassionate. Chronic pain is no joke.'[11] Gaga's 2016 album *Joanne* is written about her aunt, who died at nineteen from complications of lupus, an autoimmune condition that mainly affects women.

Selena Gomez, another American pop star, has spoken out about having lupus and how the disease impacts her life. In 2017, Gomez revealed in an Instagram post that she'd had a kidney transplant due to lupus complications and that the kidney was donated by her friend. 'Lupus continues to be very misunderstood but progress is being made,' she wrote on Instagram and advised people to visit the Lupus Research Alliance website.[12]

She's since helped raise more than $500,000 for the alliance,[13] and raised awareness of the mental health impacts of the auto-immune condition, telling *People* in 2016: 'I've discovered that anxiety, panic attacks and depression can be side effects of lupus, which can present their own challenges.'[14] The mental health aspects of autoimmune and chronic pain conditions are often overlooked by patients themselves as well as their doctors, so this kind of awareness-raising is invaluable for sufferers.

Venus Williams has spoken about her struggles to be diagnosed with the autoimmune condition, Sjögren's syndrome. She told the *New York Times* in 2011: 'The fatigue is hard to explain unless you have it. Some mornings I feel really sick, like when you don't get a lot of sleep or you have a flu or cold. I always have some level of tiredness. And the more I tried to push through it, the tougher it got.'[15]

None of these people are hysterical women who don't want to work; none are just a bit lazy and need some attention—stereotypes all too often applied to people with complex pain conditions. They have the world's attention in spite of their illnesses, not because of them and all live incredibly productive lives. But there is another reason for society to dislike them, and that's because they are taking up public space in a man's world, and what's more, they're asking for sympathy, something women are supposed to give to others rather than feel entitled to themselves. As Kate Manne explains in *Down Girl*, one of the ways in which misogyny works is to judge women by completely different standards to men in the same field.[16] According to standard power relations in a patriarchal society, women competing with men for positions of power or prestige are often met with hostility or even disgust.

When I read this part of Manne's book, I knew what she meant because I've been on the receiving end of it. I'm hardly a powerful person but as an editor who also occasionally writes opinion pieces, I am judged to be taking up a platform that should belong to a man. Since women are supposed to *give* their attention to men, not *take* it or demand it themselves, any woman in the public eye is immediately suspicious. I was called an 'attention seeker' on Twitter by numerous men after I wrote an article about sexism, in which I referred to the incident when my breast was groped by a stranger in a restaurant. One man emailed me to advise that I should have taken it as a compliment.

'You say you had your breast groped,' he wrote to me. 'The incident is obviously clear in your mind and the reason must be breast groping has been a very rare occurrence in your life.

'When I was a teenager in Britain in the 1960's such an incident would not be so clear in the mind of the average young woman (or some of the older ones) because a friendly squeeze of a breast or two was as common as a handshake and often delivered for the same reason as a handshake might be engaged in, in an informal social gathering to a casual acquaintance. A few women were upset by this but a surprising number weren't, depending how the squeeze was delivered. Regard-less of this most men who would give a breast a friendly tweak were also very protective of women and as long they were sober, well mannered.

'How times have changed. Women's liberation has made a friendly grope none-PC [*sic*] but it has also been a significant factor in the way society has developed; often for the worse.'

His email went on and on and I tweeted parts of it out in exasperation. But when I did, I was shocked by the response.

'No one wants to squeeze anything having to do with you. Your [*sic*] exaggerating . . . Again,' one man, whom I have never met, said. Another: 'This "woman" will not be happy until every last female hates every last WM [white man] on earth, & everyone's miserable like her.' And a series of tweets came from a man who said it was just 'so god damn annoying' that women have to draw attention to themselves when something bad happens to them.

As a woman, I am supposed to *take* that deprivation of my liberty; I deserved it because I failed to *give* my attention to the man who was demanding it. It didn't matter that I didn't know him and was trying to quietly enjoy a dinner with my boyfriend. He was *entitled* to my attention and my body, and I was a 'feminazi' and an 'attention seeker' for complaining about it.

I think Manne's analysis works especially well for Dunham, who is one of few female television writers and producers to have achieved international success. Manne argues that women are 'supposed to give everyone around them personal care and attention, or else they risk seeming nasty, mean, unfair and callous'. She adds: 'In general, the larger and more diverse a woman's audience or constituency, the more she will tend to be perceived as cold, distant, "out of touch", negligent, careless, and selfish, in view of these norms of feminine attentiveness. No such listening skills need be demonstrated by her male counterparts, however.'[17] On top of all her power and privilege, now Dunham has the temerity to ask for sympathy and demand better treatments for her illnesses. This is unlikely to elicit sympathy, according to Manne: 'Drawing attention to one's moral injuries in a public forum does not seem an especially good way to attract sympathetic attention, as a subordinate group member,' she writes. 'It seems liable to provoke hostility in many people, even in the most straightforward cases.'[18] I found this out all too clearly for myself, and my public position is a fraction of Dunham's. She is held to impossibly high standards, pilloried for not speaking for everyone, for being insensitive, in a way no male television producer ever has been. Even considering the mistakes she has made, it is hard to imagine a man in her position being hated quite as much for similar social infractions. Drawing attention to her illness only worsens her position in a patriarchal society.

Of course this misogyny feeds into how doctors view their female patients. We start in a position hostile to social norms in a patriarchal society by demanding attention and sometimes even sympathy for ourselves, when we are supposed to be giving these emotional goods to other people. In such a society, how do we get doctors to believe us when we say we don't want to be sick or in pain but we are? It strikes me as ever more absurd that this is still a message filtering through the medical establishment when they've spent centuries diagnosing women with similar symptoms and virtually no time at all investigating these symptoms on a biological level.

In this book, I've focused on chronic pain conditions because I have been shocked at what I've learnt—when researching endometriosis and adenomyosis—about the link between chronic pain conditions and autoimmune conditions, and their links with depression and anxiety. The conditions are all beleaguered by general ignorance but they aren't all uncommon. I don't want to say that diabetes, asthma, cancer, maternal health and reproductive rights aren't important—of course they are—but nobody needs their attention drawn to these conditions. I can't draw a full picture of women's health because, truth be told, I still don't know what it looks like. In this chapter, I'm just hoping to add pieces to the puzzle: those that are grossly neglected, discarded and hidden from view. These aren't conditions that kill us but they radically alter our opportunities to reach our full potential in life. And because treatments aren't standardised, they aren't all available in public health systems, meaning women and other people of lower socioeconomic status are often priced out of the best care available.

I could have, perhaps should have, included some other conditions: gynaecological cancers are one, Ehlers–Danlos syndrome is another, and of course polycystic ovary syndrome and adenomyosis are obvious omissions. But below I've highlighted the ten chronic pain conditions, and the autoimmune conditions with which they commonly co-occur, because of the links between them—and because, I think, these pieces might somehow fit together in the puzzle. These conditions have overlapping symptoms and similar quality of life impacts. Doctors say they are hard to diagnose because the symptoms are so generalised. But are they really so hard to diagnose when you're listening carefully?

There is very little information on some of these conditions and most of it comes from the US, where the research organisations and patient advocacy groups have begun to shine a spotlight on them. Some of the information below refers only to the US, but I have tried to include Australian and British figures where I have been able to access the information.

CHRONIC PAIN CONDITIONS

Chronic pelvic pain is a disease in its own right and should be treated as such. Endometriosis, vulvodynia, irritable bowel syndrome, painful bladder syndrome (interstitial cystitis) and pelvic muscle disorders may all be part of an overriding chronic pelvic pain condition. These conditions also have strong correlations with chronic fatigue syndrome, fibromyalgia, and chronic headaches or migraines. However, since the diseases below are still treated and funded on an individualised basis, and the overall picture of chronic pelvic pain remains unclear, I've singled them out for clarity.

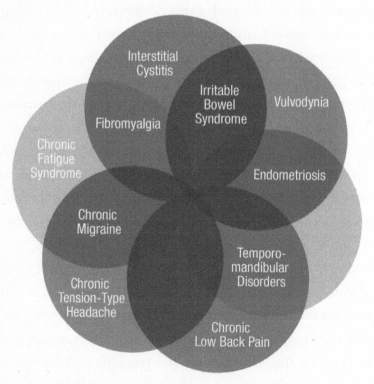

The ten chronic overlapping pain conditions
Source: Chronic Pain Research Alliance

Endometriosis

Endometriosis is a chronic inflammatory disease in which tissue similar to the lining of the uterus grows in other parts of the body, most commonly in the pelvic cavity on organs such as the ovaries, bladder, bowel and pelvic sidewall, but very occasionally in other parts of the body such as the lungs and brain. These deposits of tissue respond to the hormonal cycle and bleed, causing inflammation, scar tissue and adhesions, sometimes fusing organs together. Symptoms include pain in the abdomen, lower back and legs, painful menstruation, pain during or after sex, fatigue, bowel and/or bladder problems, bloating, nausea and heavy or irregular periods. It may also cause low mood, sleep problems, dizziness and anxiety. In some cases, it can lead to infertility.

Around one in ten women of reproductive age have endometriosis. It's the second most common gynaecological condition and has been recognised by medical science for over a century. Yet it still takes an average of seven to ten years for it to be diagnosed. A portion of the delayed diagnosis is due to women and others with female reproductive organs not seeing a doctor because they believe their pain is normal. But the majority of the delay is down to doctors dismissing period pain as normal, a poor understanding among both general practitioners and specialists about the disease, difficulty of diagnosis and a severe lack of research and focus on it.

At least 176 million women around the world have the condition, and its economic burden is huge—at least US\$119 billion annually to the US economy, A\$6.6 billion to the Australian economy and £8.2 billion to the UK economy.[19] The average annual societal cost per patient globally is US\$16,116.

Of that, the personal cost to those who have the disease is life-altering: US$13,048 in productivity lost per woman per year and US$3066 in direct healthcare costs.[20] Awareness of the condition has been growing in the past few years, but research funding hasn't improved globally and few novel treatments are currently in the pipeline. Although endo affects about the same number of women as diabetes and has a similar economic cost, it receives 5 per cent of the funding of diabetes—again, this figure is pretty constant from the US to the UK to Australia. It isn't a lifestyle disease and can't be prevented—although if diagnosed early, it can be well managed.

There's no known cause or cure. Endo currently has three treatment options: hormones, surgery or pain management. The same treatments won't work for every sufferer, so effective treatment is by trial and error. There's some evidence that skilled excision laparoscopic surgery is effective on deep-infiltrating endometriosis, but mounting evidence that multiple surgeries are ineffective and can cause more pain. An overview of Cochrane Reviews conducted by the Chronic Pain Research Alliance found low to moderate evidence for treatments and that three hormonal treatments—GnRH analogues, danazol and depot progestogens—were associated with higher rates of harm than other interventions.[21] The US NIH spent $7 million on endo research in 2014, representing US$1.11 per patient. Australia's research funding body, the National Health and Medical Research Council (NHMRC), spent A$839,695 (US$593,244) in 2017, representing A$1.20 per patient. In 2018 and 2019, $15 million in funding was announced by the Australian government for endometriosis, a potential step change in recognition and treatment for the disease.

Twenty per cent of endo sufferers also have other chronic pain conditions such as irritable bowel syndrome, interstitial cystitis/ painful bladder syndrome, vulvodynia, temporomandibular joint disorder, migraine and fibromyalgia, and/or they have autoimmune disorders such as systemic lupus erythematosus, rheumatoid arthritis, chronic fatigue syndrome and Sjögren's syndrome.[22] Another study found that hypothyroidism, fibro-myalgia, chronic fatigue syndrome, autoimmune diseases, allergies and asthma are all significantly more common in women with endo than in women in the general US population.[23]

Vulvodynia

Vulvodynia is chronic pain in the vulva without an identifiable cause. The most common symptom is a burning or stinging pain, and some sufferers report a feeling of rawness in the vulva. The pain might only occur in a very specific area of the perineum, such as the vestibulum, labia or clitoris, or it can affect the whole external genital area. Sitting, using tampons and sexual intercourse can all cause intense pain or be impos-sible for sufferers of vulvodynia. There are two types of this condition: unprovoked vulvodynia, in which the pain is spon-taneous and not triggered by pressure or contact; and provoked vulvodynia, in which the pain is triggered by touch, usually in the vestibulum and commonly from sexual intercourse, inserting tampons, tight clothing, cycling or horseriding.

One in four women of all ages and ethnicities may be affected at some point in their lives. The prevalence of clinically confirmed vulvodynia is estimated at between 3 and 7 per cent of reproductive-aged women, but it may be as high as 18 per cent, according to the International Association for the Study of Pain. The economic impact in the United States is estimated to be between US$31 and $72 billion, 70 per cent of which is direct healthcare costs. Symptoms can begin at any age but most commonly begin between the ages of eighteen and 25.[24] There are currently no FDA-approved treatments for vulvodynia. There's no known cause or cure. There's evidence of central sensitisation in vulvodynia patients[25] and that treatments used for other chronic pain syndromes may also be effective in treating vulvodynia.[26] Women with vulvodynia often have pelvic floor dysfunction so physiotherapy can be of benefit; however, professionals skilled in treatment for vulvodynia are rare.

The US National Institutes of Health (NIH) spent $3 million on the condition in 2014, representing 50 cents per patient for that year. The NHMRC devoted zero funding to vulvodynia from 2013 to 2017. Urinary or bowel disorders such as interstitial cystitis/painful bladder syndrome or irritable bowel syndrome are frequently associated with provoked vulvodynia.

Fibromyalgia

Fibromyalgia is defined as a common rheumatologic syndrome characterised by chronic, diffuse musculoskeletal pain and tenderness. In layman's terms, it's a chronic condition that causes aches and pains all over the body. As well as pain, symptoms include disturbed or unrefreshing sleep, fatigue, and cognitive and memory difficulties (sometimes called fibro fog). Nine out ten people diagnosed with fibromyalgia are women, and it most often occurs between the ages of twenty and 50. It is estimated to affect about 2 per cent of people of all genders, ages, cultures and ethnic groups, and to represent a cost of

$20 billion a year to the US healthcare system. The impact on quality of life is substantial and comparable with that of rheumatoid arthritis.[27] In the United States, about 15 per cent of patients receive state-funded disability payments due to the severity of the symptoms.[28] To be diagnosed with fibromyalgia, patients must have had a history (more than three months) of widespread pain and tenderness to eleven of eighteen tender points defined by the American College of Rheumatology,[29] although there is some disagreement about the adequacy of this diagnosis criteria. Other symptoms of fibromyalgia include short-term memory loss, headaches, light-headedness, dizziness, feeling faint, restless leg syndrome, teeth grinding during the night, morning stiffness, pelvic pain, tingling or numbness in hands and feet, and bowel and/or bladder problems.

The NIH spent $10 million on fibromyalgia research in 2014: $1.67 per patient. The NHMRC spent A$81,000 in 2017, 17 cents per patient. There are three FDA-approved treatments for fibromyalgia, but an Agency for Healthcare Research and Quality Comparative Effectiveness Review found that 'overall treatment effects were small and even less when substantial placebo-group improvements were considered'.[30]

There's no known cause or cure, although some evidence points to onset following physical or psychological trauma or severe stress, or following an infection or virus. There's evidence of central sensitisation in people with fibromyalgia. People with fibromyalgia are more likely to have depression (40 per cent), anxiety (45 per cent), irritable bowel syndrome (70 per cent), period pain, interstitial cystitis/painful bladder syndrome, autoimmune conditions including rheumatoid arthritis, lupus erythematosus and Sjögren's syndrome, chronic fatigue syndrome, myofascial pain syndrome, low back pain and temporomandibular joint disorder.[31]

Chronic fatigue syndrome/Myalgic encephalomyelitis

The US Centers for Disease Control and Prevention defines CFS/ME as 'a complex, chronic, debilitating disease . . . characterized by reduced ability to perform pre-illness activities that lasts for more than 6 months and is accompanied by profound fatigue, which is not improved by rest'.[32] Symptoms affect different parts of the body and can include unrefreshing sleep or trouble sleeping, weakness, muscle and joint pain, problems with concentration or memory, headaches, sore throats and tender lymph nodes in the neck or under the arm. Symptoms may be mild to severe. They may come and go, or they may last for weeks, months or years. They can also happen over time or come on suddenly.

Less common symptoms include blurry eyes, sensitivity to light, eye pain, mood swings, anxiety, chills and night sweats, low-grade fever or low body temperature, irritable bowel, allergies, and numbing, tingling or burning sensations in the face, hands or feet. These chronic and debilitating symptoms are known to increase long-term disability and premature death.[33]

CFS/ME affects 1 million Americans, 250,000 Britons, and between 94,000 and 242,000 Australians. Up to 17 million people worldwide have CFS/ME. Women are two to four times more likely than men to have it. The onset of symptoms usually occurs in two distinct age ranges: 10 to 19 years, then 30 to 39 years. It affects men and women, and all cultures, ethnicities and socioeconomic groups. The burden is estimated to be $37 billion annually to the US economy in medical costs and lost productivity.

There's no known cause or cure, so treatments aim to improve symptoms. There are no FDA-approved treatments, and so-called evidence-based treatments are hotly contested. Following research claiming to show that graded exercise therapy (gradually increasing the amount of exercise you do each day) was effective, this became a first-line treatment for patients around the world; later research, however, showed it actually made many patients worse.

The NIH spent $5 million on research in 2014, $1.25 per patient. The NHMRC spent A$115,438 or between 48 cents and $1.23 per person in 2017. However, in late 2017 a lobbying effort led to the NHMRC forming an expert advisory committee to direct research funds towards the most prospective areas of biomedical research, and to develop national guidelines for diagnosis and treatment. In 2018, the Australian Senate passed a unanimous motion for a unified research and advocacy effort for CFS/ME. In 2015, the US National Institute of Medicine released a major report on ME/CFS which recommended changing its name to 'systemic exertion intolerance disease', proposed new diagnostic criteria and called for more research.[34] In 2017, the NIH announced it was awarding four grants worth $7 million to establish a coordinated scientific research effort on ME/CFS. The UK's National Institute for Health and Care Excellence is currently updating its guidance on ME/CFS, which will be released in 2020.

Looking back now, I don't think I ever met the diagnostic criteria for chronic fatigue syndrome. I now recognise what I was experiencing as a typical endo flare-up. This misdiagnosis almost certainly led to the delay in my eventual diagnosis of endometriosis.

Migraine and chronic tension-type headaches

A migraine is an intense throbbing headache, usually occurring on one side of the head but sometimes on both. It's a neurological disease that affects 1 billion people worldwide, and three out of every four people who experience migraines are women. Migraines usually produce intense pain in the temples or behind one eye or ear and can also cause nausea, vomiting, and sensitivity to light and sound. The symptoms can be severely disabling and can prevent sufferers from participating in daily activities like work, home or caring duties and social activities. Migraine is the third most prevalent illness in the world and the sixth most disabling, with 90 per cent of people unable to function normally during a migraine attack. It affects children as well as adults but is often undiagnosed in children. More boys than girls experience migraine, but incidence and severity rise in girls after puberty. Up to one-third of people with migraine perceive an aura: a transient visual, sensory, language or motor disturbance.

A tension-type headache is characterised by pain that feels like pressure, tightening or a sensation like the head is being squeezed in a vice. It's often felt on both sides of the head. The pain can radiate from the lower back of the head, neck, eyes or various muscle groups.

Both migraine and tension-type headache are considered chronic when they occur 15 days or more a month for three months in the absence of medication use with migraine or for six months with tension-type headache. Between 1.4 per cent and 2.2 per cent of people experience chronic migraine, and 2.2 per cent of people experience chronic tension-type headache.[35] Both are more common in women than men.

It's believed that migraine has a genetic link, as it typically runs in families.

While research and understanding of migraine has improved dramatically in the past two decades, it's still poorly understood and often goes untreated, despite there now being clear diagnostic criteria and evidence of its effects from brain-imaging techniques. It's estimated that while a quarter of people with migraine would benefit from preventive medicine currently available, only 12 per cent receive it and more than half of all migraine sufferers go undiagnosed.

Migraine is estimated to cost the US economy $36 billion annually in healthcare and lost productivity. There are fourteen FDA-approved medications for migraine, one for chronic migraine and none for chronic tension-type headache. In 2014, the NIH spent $285,000 on chronic tension-type headache, or four cents per person, and $20 million on chronic migraine, or $2.86 per person. In total in 2015, NIH funding per person with migraine was just 50 cents per sufferer. In Australia, the NHMRC devoted A$811,494 in 2017 to migraine—that's 17 cents per person.

People with migraine are more likely to have depression, anxiety, sleep disorders, irritable bowel syndrome, fibromyalgia, restless leg syndrome, epilepsy, obesity and asthma. Research is also starting to show that people with migraine have an increased risk of heart attacks and stroke.[36]

Chronic low back pain

While low back pain is often a symptom of another condition, the NIH Task Force on Standards for Chronic Low Back Pain states that it can progress, like any other chronic pain condition, 'beyond a symptomatic state to a complex condition unto itself'.[37] Chronic low back pain occurs between the lower ribs and lower bottom at least half of the days in a six-month period. Symptoms include dull aching, sharp pain and/or tingling or burning sensations in the lower back. Some people with chronic low back pain also experience weakness in the legs or feet.

Chronic low back pain is estimated to affect about 39 per cent of people worldwide at some point in their lives, and it occurs from teenage years into old age. There's been little substantial research into this pain as a condition in itself, which makes it hard to come by figures on economic costs and the co-occurrence of this pain with other chronic pain conditions, although research from the Chronic Pain Research Alliance shows it commonly occurs with the nine other chronic pain conditions outlined here. Some studies show that chronic low back pain is more common in women than men, often caused by pregnancy-related issues. Chronic back pain overall is split evenly among men and women. There are no FDA-approved treatments specifically targeted at chronic low back pain.

The NIH spent $24 million on low back pain research in 2014—that's $1.23 per patient. I wasn't able to get figures just on low back pain from the NHMRC, although it spent A$6,309,501 on chronic back pain research in 2017.

Irritable bowel syndrome

Irritable bowel syndrome (IBS) is a collection of symptoms including abdominal pain and cramping, bloating, diarrhoea, constipation or both diarrhoea and constipation that are experienced for longer than three months in the absence of any visible disease of the gastrointestinal tract. It's estimated to affect 14 per cent of the general population. Women are twice as likely as men to have IBS, and adults under the age of 45 are more likely than older adults to suffer from it.

There's no known cause or cure for IBS, but some research suggests that symptoms may be eased with dietary changes. There are three FDA-approved treatments available for IBS; a systematic review of the twelve main treatments for IBS found low or very low evidence for nine of them.

The direct and indirect cost to the US economy of IBS may be as high as $380 billion annually. The NIH spent US$14 million on IBS in 2014, working out at 32 cents per patient. The NHMRC spent A$497,000 in 2017 or 14 cents per patient.

People with IBS are more likely to have another chronic pain condition than the general population.

Interstitial cystitis/Painful bladder syndrome

Interstitial cystitis (IC) is also known as painful bladder syndrome and bladder pain syndrome. It is pain, pressure or discomfort experienced in the bladder, in the absence of any infection or other disease, that lasts more than three months. As well as pain, symptoms include feeling the need to urinate urgently or frequently, or both, and pain during sex.

Anyone can develop IC, but it's more common in women. American studies have estimated that between 3 and 8 million women suffer from IC and 1 to 4 million men in the United States. Direct costs to the US economy have been estimated at $22 billion annually.[38] There may be a genetic link, as people with a family history of IC are more likely to suffer from it.

IC isn't the same as a urinary tract infection, but a previous infection may cause IC by damaging or irritating the bladder's lining. Sadly, very little is understood about IC, and it's difficult to get diagnosed as doctors still disagree about what it is and if it exists. However, researchers are studying whether it has an autoimmune element.

IC remains a controversial diagnosis not only among doctors but also among some patient groups. The patient advocacy group Live UTI Free, for example, claims the standard UTI test in use for almost 60 years misses up to 50 per cent of all infections; this would mean one in two women are at risk of being misdiagnosed, with significant numbers progressing from recurrent UTI to diagnoses of so-called untreatable conditions like IC. In other words, the advocacy group believes that some patients being diagnosed with IC have an infection that won't be treated once this diagnosis is given. Some doctors in the US and UK agree; they claim to have found infections undetectable in generic tests among women with recurrent UTIs, and have developed effective treatment protocols for these people. However, there are few randomised controlled studies on effective treatments for either recurrent UTIs or IC.

Some bladder pain can be caused by dysfunction in the muscles of the pelvic floor, lower abdomen or back and may improve with physiotherapy. There's one FDA-approved treatment for IC. A review of evidence for the most common treatments for IC found a majority had very little proof of efficacy. The NIH spent $9 million in 2014 on IC, working out at $1.13 per patient. The NHMRC funded no research into IC from 2013 to 2017.

Women with IC also commonly have irritable bowel syndrome, fibromyalgia, chronic fatigue syndrome, endometriosis, vulvodynia and allergies.

Temporomandibular joint disorder

Temporomandibular joint disorder (TMD) refers to a common condition characterised by pain in the jaw joint and surrounding muscles and tissues. Symptoms include jaw and face pain, difficulty speaking, chewing, swallowing and making facial expressions. In severe cases, patients may have trouble breathing.

Signs of TMD appear in up to 60 to 70 per cent of the global population, although only 5 to 12 per cent receives treatment.[39] Women are four times more likely than men to suffer from TMD.[40] Symptoms most often begin between the ages of twenty and 40. Ninety per cent of people seeking treatment for TMD are women of reproductive age.[41]

There are no FDA-approved treatments for TMD. Two reviews examining the effectiveness of the drugs most commonly used to treat TMD-related pain couldn't find evidence either way, meaning it's unknown how well these treatments work.

TMD has been estimated to cost the US economy $32 billion a year. The NIH funded $18 million worth of research on TMD in 2014, or 51 cents per patient. The NHMRC funded no research on the condition between 2013 and 2017.

People with TMD are more likely to have another chronic pain condition. People with TMD who also have migraine and/or fibromyalgia report greater pain intensity and duration of TMD.[42]

AUTOIMMUNE CONDITIONS

Autoimmune diseases are conditions in which the body's immune system, which defends the body against bacteria, viruses and other germs, turns on itself and starts to attack its own healthy cells, tissues and/or organs. We know of about a hundred autoimmune conditions, and they range in severity according to where they occur in the body. Around 5 to 8 per cent of the population is affected, and three-quarters of those affected are women. It isn't known why women are more susceptible to autoimmune conditions, although the disparity has been known for well over a hundred years. Only this century has attention started to focus on the sex and gender difference. The basic immune response between men and women is different: women produce a more vigorous immune response and make more antibodies. When men contract autoimmune conditions, they tend to be more severe than in women.[43]

In *Inferior*, Angela Saini noted that one of the reasons for women's greater susceptibility to autoimmune conditions is that 'women's immune systems are so powerful that they can sometimes backfire'. She cites Kathryn Sandberg, the director of the Georgetown University Center for the Study of Sex Differences in Health, Aging and Disease, as saying, 'You start regarding yourself as foreign, and your immune system starts attacking its own cells.' Sandberg elaborates: 'It's kind of a double-edged sword with the immune system. In some ways it's better to have a female immune system if you're fighting off infection of any kind, but on the other hand, we are more susceptible to autoimmune diseases, which are very problematic.'[44]

Autoimmune conditions are a leading cause of death and disability in women around the world. There's some evidence of a genetic link in autoimmune conditions since they appear to run in families, although not all family members may be affected by the same autoimmune condition. As well as genetics, environmental exposure—such as to a virus, bacteria, toxin or sunlight—may trigger autoimmune conditions.

Much is still unknown about autoimmune conditions. Some of the more well-known or common ones include type 1 diabetes, Crohn's disease, multiple sclerosis, rheumatoid arthritis, psoriasis, thyroiditis and lupus. Although each condition has its own symptoms, most autoimmune conditions cause fatigue, dizziness and low-grade fever. In most, but not all, symptoms can come and go and—similar to those of chronic pain conditions—can flare up at times, producing more intense and severe symptoms. It's hard to get statistics on research funding for specific autoimmune conditions, but the NIH reports that it devoted $934 million to autoimmune diseases in 2017. The NHMRC couldn't provide a total figure on funding it granted for autoimmune conditions but it did provide figures for funding for lupus, Graves' disease and Sjögren's syndrome, which I have included below.

The autoimmune conditions I've outlined here frequently co-occur with other chronic pain conditions, and are more prevalent in women than men.

Lupus

Systemic lupus erythematosus (SLE or, simply, lupus) is a chronic autoimmune disease that can damage the joints, skin, kidneys, heart, lungs and other parts of the body. Its symptoms vary from person to person but include fatigue, fever, weight loss, hair loss, mouth sores, butterfly rash across the nose and cheeks, rashes on other parts of the body, painful or swollen joints and muscle pain, sensitivity to the sun, chest pain, headaches, dizziness, seizure, memory problems, or changes in behaviour. Nine out of ten adults with systemic lupus erythematosus are female, and symptoms range from mild to severe.

There are other types of lupus: cutaneous lupus erythematosus, also known as discoid lupus, which affects only the skin; drug-induced lupus, caused by certain drugs used to treat other chronic health problems; and neonatal lupus, a rare condition in infants caused by certain antibodies passed from the mother. SLE is the most common and severe form of lupus.

While anyone can get lupus, it is more common and more severe in women of African, Asian, Indigenous and Polynesian heritage in Australia, the US and UK. Although it's more common than leukaemia and multiple sclerosis, it's considered a rare disease, and poor record keeping means accurate figures on sufferers are hard to come by. However, it's estimated that at least 5 million people worldwide have a form of lupus, mostly women of reproductive age. In Australia, Indigenous people are two to four times more likely (and probably more) to have lupus than other Australians, and it has higher rates of premature death and disability in Indigenous Australians compared to other Australians. The reasons for this aren't known, but access to quality healthcare is a major issue for Indigenous Australians and that probably plays a role. A similar pattern of disease severity exists among women of colour in the US and UK.

Accurate and well-sourced figures on lupus funding and costs are also hard to come by. However, a 2008 study published in *Arthritis and Rheumatology* found that the average direct and lost productivity costs in the US were around US$20,000 per patient per year.[45] The NHMRC spent just over $2.5 million on lupus research in 2018.

Women who have lupus are at higher risk than other women of heart disease, osteoporosis and kidney disease. One in three lupus patients suffers from one or more other auto-immune conditions, and it's common for people with lupus to suffer from depression. They may also have low testosterone. Ten to 15 per cent of lupus patients die prematurely due to complications of the condition, but it can be well managed with specialist care and early diagnosis. The delay in diagnosis of lupus is between six and seven years, and 63 per cent of lupus sufferers report being misdiagnosed. More than half of these people had to see four or more different healthcare providers in order to receive a correct diagnosis. People with lupus report pain and fatigue as the most difficult symptoms to cope with.[46]

Rheumatoid arthritis

Rheumatoid arthritis (RA) is a chronic autoimmune disease that causes pain and swelling in the joints. It happens when the immune system attacks the lining of the joints, leading to pain and inflammation and, in some cases, permanent joint damage. It usually starts in the small joints of the hands and feet but can progress to the larger joints and other body systems including the skin, eyes, heart, lungs, bone marrow and blood vessels. It usually affects joints on both sides of the body, unlike some other kinds of arthritis. Symptoms include painful, warm, swollen and/or aching joints; joint stiffness that's worse in the morning or after a period of inactivity; fatigue; fever; weight loss; muscle pain and depression.

Rheumatoid arthritis is the most common rheumatic auto-immune condition and the most severe form of arthritis. It affects roughly 1 per cent of the global population—or about 1.3 million people in the US,[47] about 408,000 in Australia[48] and more than 400,000 in the UK.[49] It occurs in all races and ethnic groups. Three-quarters of people with RA are women, and it usually begins during their reproductive years. For men, it usually develops later in life and tends to be more severe. There's no known cause, although—as in all autoimmune conditions—genetic and environmental factors are believed to play a role. Smoking increases the risk of developing RA and increases the severity of symptoms.

RA can be effectively treated with specialised care, and due to advances in pharmaceutical treatments fewer people today become disabled from RA. However, there's no single diagnostic test, and because joint swelling and stiffness can be caused by many conditions there's sometimes a delay in diagnosis. A specialist doctor called a rheumatologist usually makes the diagnosis—the earlier, the better and more effective treatment will be. In 2017 the NIH spent $93 million on RA research.

People with RA are at higher risk of developing osteoporosis, heart disease, lung disease, lymphoma and infections. Half of people with RA also have Sjögren's syndrome. Depression is common among people with RA.

Sjögren's syndrome

Sjögren's (pronounced *SHOW-grins*) syndrome is an auto-immune condition that attacks the mucus-producing glands of the body, most often those that produce tears and saliva, but it can also affect the mucous membranes in the nose and vagina. Its most common features are dry eyes, dry mouth and fatigue. Eyes can burn, itch or feel gritty; they may be sensitive to light, and eyelids may stick together. The mouth can feel so dry that it's difficult for them to swallow or speak, while the mouth and tongue may have a burning sensation, and tooth decay is common. Other symptoms may include vaginal dryness, joint pain, swollen salivary glands, skin rashes, dry skin and persistent dry cough. Oral thrush, a bacterial overgrowth in the mouth, may also develop.

Ninety per cent of sufferers are women, and it's most common between the ages of 40 and 50. Global prevalence rates on this condition are hard to come by, although it's estimated to affect about 0.5 to 1 per cent of the global population.[50] It often goes undiagnosed when all symptoms aren't considered together. A dentist may treat dry mouth and dental decay and not know about the eye or vaginal dryness. Some women are told it's just a symptom of menopause that will pass. An ophthalmologist treating dry eyes may not enquire about or consider dry mouth, fatigue and other symptoms. The average delay in diagnosis is six years.[51]

Rheumatologists have primary responsibility for diagnosing people with this disease, although they may refer to other health professionals for the treatment of symptoms. There are a number of prescription and over-the-counter medications that can treat the symptoms of Sjögren's syndrome.

About half of people with Sjögren's also have rheumatoid arthritis and/or lupus. They may have low testosterone. They may also be diagnosed with fibromyalgia or chronic fatigue syndrome/ME, and it can be unclear whether or not the diagnosis is mistaken because of the similarity of the symptoms. They can be at increased risk of developing cardiovascular disease and cancers such as lymphoma. Less commonly, Sjögren's can cause lung, kidney and liver damage. Some sufferers may also develop numbness, tingling or burning in their hands and feet, known as peripheral neuropathy. They often also have depression.

The NHMRC spent almost $288,000 on Sjögren's syndrome research in 2018, a big jump from $81,000 in 2017.

Thyroid diseases (Hashimoto's thyroiditis and Graves' disease)
The most common autoimmune diseases occur in the thyroid, a small butterfly-shaped gland at the base of the neck, just

below the Adam's apple. It produces the thyroid hormone, which travels through the body and controls its metabolism, including how fast calories are burnt and how fast the heart beats. Hashimoto's thyroiditis is the most common form of *hypo*thyroidism, in which the thyroid is underactive and doesn't produce enough thyroid hormones. It affects 1 to 2 per cent of people, and ten times more women than men. Graves' disease is a type of *hyper*thyroidism resulting from an overactive thyroid, which produces more hormones than the body needs. It affects five times as many women as men. Both Hashimoto's and Graves' can lead to infertility and miscarriage, but their potential to do this can be reversed with treatment. Both conditions can improve during pregnancy but become worse in the year after giving birth.

In Hashimoto's thyroiditis, the immune system makes antibodies known as T cells that attack the thyroid gland, interfering with the production of hormones. The most common symptoms are weight gain, feeling cold, poor concentration and depression. Other symptoms include fatigue, constipation, dry skin, hair loss, heavy and irregular periods, and an enlarged thyroid called a goitre. Some people have no symptoms for a long time. Hypothyroidism can cause miscarriage and birth defects, so it's essential that it's treated during pregnancy: this is easily done by taking tablets to replace the thyroid hormones the body isn't producing. But it can take a while to get the levels right; constant monitoring is required.

In Graves' disease, the immune system makes antibodies that attack the receptors for thyroid-stimulating hormone, leading it to produce too much thyroid hormone. The most common symptoms are bulging eyes, weight loss and a fast metabolism.

Other symptoms include heart palpitations or rapid pulse; thickening and reddening of the skin, especially on the shins and upper feet; irritability or nervousness; feeling hot, flushed and/or sweating; fatigue; muscle weakness; trouble sleeping; shaky hands; diarrhoea or increased bowel movements; and goitre, which can make the neck look swollen. Hyperthyroidism can cause sufferers to feel very energetic, but the increased heart rate and pulse may also make people with the condition feel jumpy or irritable. About half of women with Graves' disease develop eye inflammation, leading to protruding eyes and impaired vision or eye irritation. Graves' can be well managed with medication or sometimes surgery to remove the gland or part of it, or radioactive iodine to destroy thyroid tissue. Untreated, it can lead to heart problems, osteoporosis, and issues in pregnancy for mother and foetus.

Hashimoto's thyroiditis and Graves' disease commonly co-occur with rheumatoid arthritis and lupus. As in many autoimmune diseases, these can also co-occur with fibromyalgia and/or chronic fatigue syndrome/ME. Many people with type 1 diabetes develop Hashimoto's thyroiditis, and people with Hashimoto's have a slightly higher risk of developing a form of thyroid cancer.

In 2018, the NHMRC spent $411,000 on Graves' disease research but nothing on Hashimoto's thyroiditis.

I find it extremely hard to believe that the co-occurrence of these diseases can be just a coincidence. As Susan Evans says, here is an area ripe for disruption. Who's ready to disrupt?

CHAPTER 8

'Ripe for disruption': why medical science must improve its knowledge of women

From the earliest days of medicine, women have been considered inferior versions of men. In *On the Generation of Animals*, the Greek philosopher Aristotle characterised a female as a mutilated male, and this belief has persisted in Western medical culture.[1] 'For much of documented history women have been excluded from medical and science knowledge production, so essentially we've ended up with a healthcare system, among other things in society, that has been made by men for men,' Dr Kate Young tells me. Historically, she says, men have made 'the medical science about women and their bodies, and there is an abundance of research evidence about the ways in which that knowledge has been constructed to reinforce the hysteria discourse and women as reproductive bodies discourse. One of my favourite examples is that in some of the first sketches of skeletons, male anatomy artists intentionally made women's hips look wider and their craniums look much smaller as a way of saying, here is our evidence that women are reproductive bodies and they need to stay at home and we can't risk making them infertile by making them too educated, look how tiny their heads are. And we see that again and again.'

Not only have doctors, scientists and researchers mostly been men, but most of the cells, animals and humans studied in medical science have also been male: most of the advances we've seen in medicine have come from the study of male biology. Dr Janine Austin Clayton, associate director for women's health research at the United States National Institutes of Health, told the *New York Times* that the result is,

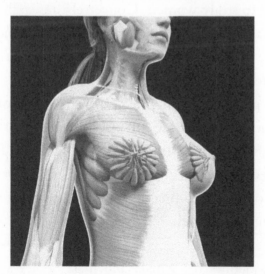

This image went viral when posted online in 2019—we are so unused to seeing women's bodies represented scientifically.
Source: Shubangi Ganeshrao Kene / Getty

'We literally know less about every aspect of female biology compared to male biology.'[2]

Medicine has always seen women first and foremost as reproductive bodies. Our reproductive organs were the greatest source of difference to men—and because they were different, they were mysterious and suspicious. But the fallout of this difference is that for a long time medicine assumed it was the *only* difference. Because women had reproductive organs, they should reproduce, and all else about them was deemed uninteresting.

In the early twentieth century, the endocrine system—which produces hormones—was discovered. To medical minds, this represented another difference between men and women, over-taking the uterus as the primary perpetrator of all women's ills. Still, medicine persisted with the belief that all other organs and functions would operate the same in men and women, so there was no need to study women. Conversely, researchers said that the menstrual cycle—and varied release of hormones through-out the cycle in rodents—introduced too many variables into a study, therefore females couldn't be studied.

Diseases presenting differently in women are often missed or misdiagnosed, and those affecting mainly women remain largely a mystery: understudied, undertreated and frequently misdiagnosed or undiagnosed. This has major knock-on effects for both medical practice and the health of women.

As Young has argued:

Medicine defines the female and male bodies as distinct but not equal; analysis of medical texts throughout history reveals the male body to be constructed as superior and the template against which bodies are judged. Any aspect of the female body that differs from the male or that cannot be given a male comparative (exemplified by the uterus) is viewed as evidence of deviation or 'fault'. Because women can bear children, medical discourse associated women with the body and men with the mind, a binary division that reinforces and is reinforced by the public–private division . . . In addition to restricting women's public contribution, such beliefs provide medicine with an explanatory model of disease and illness in women: to deny one's 'biological destiny' is to incite all manner of diseases, as Plato stated when theorising the wandering womb.[3]

We see this in many predominantly female conditions: women with endometriosis are told that delayed childbearing caused the illness, or that pregnancy will cure it; women with breast cancer were once fed this line until advances in research (which only occurred because women campaigned for better knowledge and treatments) proved otherwise.

During the 1980s, a group of female scientists in the United States formed a society to campaign for better health research in women, now called the Society for Women's Health Research. They teamed up with some US Congress members in order to draw attention to the discrepancies in medical research and the effect on women's health. A 1985 report by the Public Health Service Task Force on Women's Health warned that 'the historical lack of research focus on women's health concerns has compromised the quality of health information available to women as well as the health care they receive'.[4] The campaign drew attention to some of the absurdities that resulted from this male bias, which Maya Dusenbery has beautifully summarised in *Doing Harm*. She notes that in the early 1960s:

> observing that women tended to have lower rates of heart disease until their estrogen levels dropped after menopause, researchers conducted the first trial to look at whether supplementation with the hormone was an effective preventive treatment. The study enrolled 8341 men and no women . . . And an NIH-supported pilot study from Rockefeller University that looked at how obesity affected breast and uterine cancer didn't enrol a single woman.[5]

And that's not all.

> The Baltimore Longitudinal Study of Aging, which began in 1958 and purported to explore 'normal human aging', didn't enrol any women for the first twenty years it ran. The Physicians' Health Study, which had recently concluded that taking a daily aspirin may reduce the risk of heart disease? Conducted in 22,071 men and zero women. The 1982 Multiple Risk Factor Intervention Trial—known, aptly enough, as MRFIT—which looked at whether dietary change and exercise could help prevent heart disease: just 13,000 men.[6]

The result of this male bias in research extends beyond clinical practice. Of the ten prescription drugs taken off the market by the FDA between 1997 and 2000 due to severe adverse effects, eight caused greater health risks in women. A 2018 study found this was a result of 'serious male biases in basic, preclinical, and clinical research'.[7]

The campaign had an effect: in 1993, the US Food and Drug Administration and the National Institutes of Health mandated the inclusion of women in clinical trials. Between the 1970s and 1990s, these organisations and many other national and international regulators had a policy that ruled out women of so-called childbearing potential from early-stage drug trials. The reasoning went like this: since women are born with all the eggs they'll ever produce, they should be excluded from drug trials in case the drug proves toxic and impedes their ability to reproduce in the future. The result was that all women were excluded from trials, regardless of their age, gender status, sexual orientation, or wish or ability to bear children. Men, on the other hand, constantly reproduce their sperm, meaning they represent a reduced risk. It sounds like a sensible policy, except it treats all women like walking wombs and has introduced a huge bias into the health of the human race.

In their 1994 book *Outrageous Practices*, Leslie Laurence and Beth Weinhouse wrote: 'It defies logic for researchers to acknowledge gender difference by claiming women's hormones can affect study results—for instance, by affecting drug metabolism—but then to ignore these differences, study only men, and extrapolate the results to women.'[8]

Since the 1990s, more women have been included in clinical trials but researchers have not always analysed results by sex and/or gender. And though clinical studies have changed substantially, preclinical studies remained focused on male cell lines and male animals. A 2010 study by Annaliese Beery and Irving Zucker reviewed sex bias in research on mammals in ten biological fields during 2009 and their historical precedents. It found:

Male bias was evident in 8 disciplines and most prominent in neuroscience, with single-sex studies of male animals outnumbering those of females 5.5 to 1. In the past half-century, male bias in non-human studies has increased while declining in human studies. Studies of both sexes frequently fail to analyze results by sex. Underrepresentation of females in animal models of disease is also commonplace, and our understanding of female biology is compromised by these deficiencies.[9]

The study also found the justification that researchers gave for excluding female animals—that it introduced too much variability in results—to be 'without foundation'.

It took until 2014 for the NIH to begin to acknowledge the problem of male bias in preclinical trials, and until 2016 to mandate that any research money it granted must include female animals.

These policies and practices have often been framed as paternalistic, designed to protect women against the harmful effects of medical research. But history belies this notion. The practice of brutal experimentation of medical treatments on women extends beyond the history of hysteria.

EXPERIMENTS ON WOMEN

The American physician Dr J. Marion Sims earned his reputation as the father of modern gynaecology by developing a technique to repair vesicovaginal fistula—he operated, without anaesthesia, on a group of enslaved African-American women, whom he kept in a small hospital behind his house in Alabama between 1845 and 1849.

Obstetric fistula is a complication of obstructed childbirth in which vaginal tissue dies after prolonged pressure from the foetus, forming a hole between the vaginal canal and other organs, most often the bladder (called vesicovaginal fistula) and the rectum (rectovaginal fistula). This causes urinary and faecal incontinence. Fistula is a devastating condition and can condemn affected women to a very poor quality of life, with some even becoming outcast from their communities. It was a common childbirth injury in the nineteenth century and still is today in some parts of the developing world.

No doubt Sims' technique has saved and restored dignity to the lives of millions of women. He also invented the modern speculum—the instrument used to open the vaginal canal for examination—and the Sims position for rectal exams. But this is no defence for the ethical standards of his practice. One woman—whom we know only by her first name, Anarcha—had a particularly severe vesicovaginal fistula and a rectovaginal fistula, and was operated on 30 times without anaesthesia before the technique was perfected. Those doctors who continue to defend Sims never seem to point to the countless advances made in medical science without performing painful surgery on enslaved human beings.

His defenders also excuse his practices by noting he was a man of his time. No doubt he was. In the context of nineteenth century medicine, there seems little honour in being ordained the father of gynaecology—after all, who were his competitors operating at the time? The Englishman Isaac Baker Brown, who surgically removed the clitorises of thousands of women as a cure for insanity, epilepsy and hysteria?[10] Or American surgeon Robert Battey, who removed the healthy ovaries of thousands of women for a variety of non-gynaecological ills? No doubt some of their patients gave consent; for many more, consent was doubtful and they were often submitted to these procedures by their husbands or male relatives. But at least Battey operated with anaesthesia, and neither perfected their techniques on enslaved women.

But unethical treatment of women of colour and women of low socioeconomic backgrounds in America didn't end there. A 1927 Supreme Court decision in *Buck v. Bell* protected the state's right to compulsorily sterilise the 'unfit', 'for the protection and health of the state'.[11] In the decades that followed, more than 60,000 people were sterilised across the United States, mostly women deemed intellectually unfit to be mothers. As Mike McRae noted in *Unwell*, 'Being poor, black, indigenous or an immigrant often meant someone was more likely to be found to be unfit.'[12] Even after these eugenic sterilisation laws fell out of favour in the United States, women of colour were still being subjected to forced sterilisations—or at least sterilisations with dubious consent procedures. In southern states, some African-American women consented to tubal ligation or hysterectomies on threat of losing welfare payments; others were simply given hysterectomies without their consent while being operated on for other conditions. McRae wrote: 'In 1961, the civil-rights leader Fannie Lou Hamer was subjected to what she called "Mississippi appendectomy" when, without her consent, she was given a hysterectomy while having minor surgery to remove a tumour. "In the North Sunflower County Hospital," Hamer explained to an audience in Washington DC, "I would say about six of the ten Negro women that go to the hospital are sterilised with the tubes tied."'[13]

In 1975, the Chicago Committee to End Sterilization Abuse reported an acting director of Obstetrics and Gynaecology at a New York hospital as saying: 'In most major teaching hospitals in New York City, it is the unwritten policy to do elective hysterectomies on poor, Black and Puerto Rican women with minimal indications, to train residents . . . at least 10 per cent of gynaecological surgery in New York is done on that basis. And 99 per cent of this is done on Blacks and Puerto Rican women.'[14]

It's worth noting that the birth control movement in the United States began chiefly as a campaign to control the population among poor, black and immigrant communities. And vestiges of these ideas linger on. One woman of low socioeconomic status in Dr Kate Young's study on women's experiences of healthcare for endometriosis had a Mirena IUD inserted without her consent following a laparoscopy. This occurred in 21st-century Melbourne.

In a 2018 *Bioethics* journal article, Phoebe Friesen disabused anyone of the idea that medicine is finally free of ethically questionable behaviour towards female patients. Friesen's article documents the current practice in the US and UK (and probably other nations) for medical students to routinely perform pelvic examinations on anaesthetised women without their consent. While the custom has been outlawed in four US states and is roundly frowned upon in official documents, surveys show it's still widespread. A 2005 survey at the University of Oklahoma found 'that a large majority of medical students had given pelvic exams to gynecologic surgery patients who were under anesthesia, and that in nearly three quarters of these cases the women had not consented to the exam'.[15] A 2003 UK survey published in the *British Medical Journal* said students anonymously reported that 'at least 24 per cent of intimate examinations they performed on anesthetized patients occurred without any consent and that "on many occasions, more than one student examined the same patient"'.[16] The authors of that study wrote: 'It is worth noting that I have found no evidence or discussion of similar teaching opportunities (e.g. rectal examinations) taking place on men who are under anaesthetic, although of course, that does not necessarily mean they do not take place.'[17]

But a 2011 study across three medical schools in England, Wales and Australia found that med students were still performing pelvic examinations on female patients without their consent as well as rectal examinations on male and female patients without consent, despite school policies against the practice. While many of the students interviewed for these studies expressed concerns about the ethics of the practice, they felt they had no choice given the hierarchical nature of medicine and the culture of training. Disturbingly, others expressed no concern at all; one Australian student expressed 'no qualms' about performing an anal examination on an anaesthetised woman because she didn't think the patient's consent was relevant. Of the students asked to perform intimate examinations without patient consent, 82 per cent obeyed orders.[18]

Looked at from this angle, medicine's unwillingness to include women in scientific studies seems a lot less like magnanimous paternalism. Rather, we're left with the impression that women aren't interesting enough for scientific endeavour but good enough for practice.

MASSIVE UNDERINVESTMENT IN PAIN

This lack of scientific interest in women extends beyond clinical trials for new drugs. Medicine knows very little about conditions that mainly affect women—and doesn't seem to be on a path to correct this. Over the past decade, an increasing recognition has grown of the burden of pain on society. The 2011 report *Relieving Pain in America* put the cost at over US$500 billion and drew attention to the fact that in spite of this massive burden on life and the economy, the NIH had dedicated just $400 million to the study of pain. Chronic pain is as prevalent as cancer, heart disease and diabetes combined, yet in 2014, the NIH spent 95 per cent less on chronic pain research than research on these other conditions.[19]

In 2010, the Australian government convened a National Pain Summit that resulted in its National Pain Strategy. The strategy noted that 'Pain is Australia's third most costly health problem and arguably the developed world's largest "undiscovered" health priority.'[20] It found that less than 10 per cent of people with non-cancer chronic pain gain access to effective treatment. Another study put the cost of chronic pain to the economy at $34 billion per annum (of which a little over half is borne by people in pain) but estimated that applying evidence-based treatments could save half that: $17 billion a year. The chief medical officer of Great Britain used his 2008 annual report to highlight the extent of chronic pain in the community and the impact it has on people with pain, their families and the economy at large. After the success of the Australian Pain Summit in raising awareness of the issues and developing a national strategy, Britain followed suit with its own pain summit in 2011. It found 7.8 million Britons were living with chronic pain, half of whom were depressed, and that this cost the economy £5 to £10 billion in lost productivity. Almost half the people living with pain—46 per cent—had three or more other long-term conditions, making them hard to treat.[21]

All three reports from the US, Australia and the UK recognised the need for improved information on chronic pain, and the lack of education in medical schools and lack of training for medical professionals in treating pain. They also recognised the lack of public awareness of pain as a serious disease state and the social stigma involved. In all nations, chronic pain correlates with economic disadvantage. While some improvements have been made to raise awareness among both health professionals and the public of chronic pain as a disease state, only very recently have the roles of sex and gender in this pain been raised as pressing issues.

Way back in 2007, pain researchers were drawing attention to this issue by publishing a consensus report on sex and gender differences in pain and analgesia. The study, published in *Pain* journal, found that

at least 79 per cent of animal studies published in *Pain* over the preceding 10 years included male subjects only, with a mere 8 per cent of studies on females only, and another 4 per cent explicitly designed to test for sex differences (the rest did not specify). Given the substantially greater prevalence of many clinical pain conditions in women vs. men, and growing evidence for sex differences in sensitivity to experimental pain and to analgesics, we recommend that all pain researchers consider testing their hypotheses in both sexes, or if restricted by practical considerations, only in females.[22]

The authors added: 'It is invalid to assume that data obtained in male subjects will generalize to females, and the best non-human model of the modal human pain sufferer—a woman—is a female animal.'[23] Pain research on women and female animals has definitely grown in the past decade but it's clear we've got a lot of catching up to do.

While the pain policies have focused on cancer pain, paediatric pain, pain in the elderly and arthritic pain, there's been very little mention to date of the huge burden of pain suffered by women in the prime of their lives, or the pain girls endure through their teenage years when they're setting up the foundations for the rest of their lives. The *Pelvic Pain Report* notes the conundrum of governments placing increased importance on chronic and complex health conditions—while, at the same time, consistently overlooking chronic pelvic pain, which it describes as 'one of the most prevalent conditions affecting women and girls in their formative and productive years'.[24] It used endometriosis, one of the more common conditions associated with persistent pelvic pain, as an example: 'It is estimated to affect 176 million women worldwide in the 15–49 age group, which outnumbers the number of people in that age category affected by breast cancer, prostate cancer, diabetes I and II and AIDS.'[25] The report describes the significant disruption to quality of life caused by chronic pelvic pain, and the major downstream problems for individuals, families, communities, health and welfare services, and facilities and workplace productivity: 'The extent of the problem escalates dramatically if data from other pelvic pain-related conditions are included. Delays in early intervention and diagnosis create unnecessary far-reaching problems. Current services are at best fragmentary and piecemeal, and there is a large gap between best evidence and practice.'[26] In spite of this, chronic pelvic pain conditions aren't acknowledged or included in the Australian government's policies and reports on women's health, chronic conditions, young people in Australia, Indigenous Australians, or rural and remote health strategies. The 2010 National Pain Strategy didn't mention chronic pelvic pain or any of its associated conditions. A 2003 Australian government report on the health and wellbeing of young people[27] listed asthma, diabetes and cancers as key priority conditions, and describes factors such as obesity that contribute to this risk. The report presents clear evidence prioritising these conditions, yet the prevalence of endometriosis and pelvic pain data equals or surpasses that of these conditions.[28]

Pelvic pain frequently affects young women, often from their early teens, and we now know this can set them up for chronic pain conditions in later life. However, paediatric pelvic pain is poorly researched, and associated health conditions such as endometriosis frequently aren't considered in determining the cause of the pain or providing age-appropriate health interventions in this group.

There's also a growing awareness in the research community of the propensity for people, particularly women, to develop further chronic pain conditions once they have one, and we saw in the last chapter how these commonly co-occur with autoimmune conditions and mental health issues.

The US Chronic Pain Research Alliance estimated in a 2015 report that chronic overlapping pain conditions affect more than 50 million American women who consume upwards of $80 billion annually in direct and indirect healthcare expenses. Yet federal investment in researching these conditions amounted to just $1.06 per patient in 2014, down 8 per cent on the previous year. A similar situation exists in Australia. The National Health and Medicine Research Council told me they invested $0 in temporomandibular joint disorder (affecting between 1.2 million and 2.9 million Australians); $0 in chronic pelvic pain (affecting about 2.4 million); $0 in vulvodynia (affecting between 1.2 million and 2.4 million Australians); and $0 in painful bladder syndrome or interstitial cystitis (at least 64,000) in the years from 2013 to 2017. In 2017, it spent a total of $8.7 million on chronic fatigue syndrome, chronic back pain, irritable bowel syndrome, migraine, endometriosis and fibromyalgia combined.[29] The figures for how many people are affected by these chronic pain conditions are extremely hard to come by because there's so little information about them. But using the most conservative estimates for how many Australians suffer from these conditions, it seems the NHMRC spent 59 cents per sufferer in 2017. Compare this to asthma, which received $13 million in funding in 2017 and affects 2.5 million Australians (about the same number affected by chronic pelvic pain)—that's $5.20 per sufferer. Asthma can be a debilitating condition and deserves the research funding, but how can the discrepancy be justified?

As the Chronic Pain Research Alliance noted in its 2015 report, 'As a result of the meager federal, private and industry research investment in COPCs to date, evidence-based treatment options are woefully few and inadequate.'[30] Where good treatment options exist, few people are able to access them. Without quality, evidence-based internationally agreed guidelines, doctors around the world are forced to use off-label treatments on a trial-and-error basis in order to find relief for patients with these conditions—often treatments that have little safety or efficacy data, especially when combined. The report outlines the urgent need for more systematic research into these conditions, since mounting research points to the common underlying disease mechanisms, mainly in the immune, neural and endocrine systems:

> Cumulatively, evidence suggests that the delay in accurate diagnosis and effective treatment commonly experienced by individuals with COPCs can have serious consequences, including worsening of both site-specific and body-wide symptoms, which in turn, makes COPCs more difficult to effectively treat; a vicious cycle ensues, leading to poorer health outcomes, diminished quality of life and increased disability. A wealth of studies demonstrate the profound impact these stigmatizing disorders have on all aspects of health and quality of life, putting patients at increased risk of suicide . . . The toll extends far beyond the affected and their families, substantially impacting the health, workforce and productivity of our nation as a whole.[31]

With the paltry amount of research funding committed to these conditions, the future doesn't look bright for their sufferers. As it stands, for these ten conditions there are currently 23 FDA-approved pharmaceutical treatments, sixteen of which are for migraine, and none is indicated for more than one condition. According to a systematic review of treatment efficacy conducted by the Chronic Pain Research Alliance, apart from migraine drugs, there was no good evidence that any of these treatments were very good at limiting symptoms or improving quality of life.

Relieving Pain in America reported that from 2005 to 2009, only a few of the nearly one hundred new FDA-approved drugs were for chronic pain conditions, specifically arthritis and fibromyalgia. Added to that, other than a capsaicin patch for postherpetic neuralgia,[32] no new therapeutic agents have been approved that represent truly novel approaches to pain management:

> Instead, most drugs approved recently are variations on existing molecules (e.g., pregabalin, duloxetine, nonsteroidal anti-inflammatory agents) or repackaged existing molecules (e.g., the many versions of extended-release opioids). It is ironic and concerning that 'many major pharmaceutical companies are leaving the pain market', despite the growing need for more diverse pain products and an increasing population of people with serious pain conditions.[33]

If pharmaceutical companies are leaving the pain market, not showing signs or intentions of developing new pain treatments, it's clear that research money will have to come from government bodies prioritising the understanding of pain.

A great example of the importance of government-funded research is what happened with hormone replacement therapy (HRT). At the turn of the century about a third of menopausal women in Western nations were taking HRT despite the lack of good-quality, long-term evidence for its benefits. During the 1990s, feminists pushed hard for government research into HRT after a series of scandals had provoked continued changes to the formula in the 1970s and 1980s. The government-funded

2002 Women's Health Institute study upended the industry, showing risks outweighed benefits in many cases. The number of women now using HRT is closer to 12 per cent.

Given the individual nature of chronic pain syndromes, personalised medical therapies are likely to be the best course of action—but one in which there's little incentive for pharmaceutical companies to invest, given the cost involved. But the figures above show government isn't investing either.

The US Institute of Medicine notes: 'The appreciation that pain can become a chronic disease in and of itself through aberrant activity of the central nervous system should curtail the search for underlying disease pathology and redirect treatment efforts toward the malfunctioning nervous system itself—a "mechanism-based therapeutic approach" rather than a "strictly symptom-based approach".[34]

Why it doesn't get funded

The lack of research money and attention going into chronic pain is of great concern to people working in the field. Evans tells me that in every lecture she gives to med school students, she tells them that chronic pelvic pain 'is ripe for disruption'. In many disease states, so much is already known, and research is focused on improving treatments. But in pelvic pain and other chronic pain conditions, we don't even know the true mechanism of the disease.

Evans tells me she's seen many excellent research proposals submitted to the National Health and Medical Research Council that continually fail to receive funds. While competition is tight—only 19 per cent[35] of proposals were successful in 2017—there are bigger issues at play.

All over the world, funding bodies want to support research that promises specific, measurable results. But so little is known about the mechanisms of pain that producing specific measurable results is hard. 'Research and funding are so competitive these days that in order to actually get a research project up, it has to not only be a good idea but . . . you can ascertain who your sample population is, who are all fairly similar, you can do an intervention, you can measure how successful it's been,' says Evans. 'You have a whole group of women with endo and pelvic pain—or just pelvic pain without endo—they're all different, there's no measurable anything, it's just, "how do you feel?"' As a result, she says, 'it just never gets over the line of being a reasonable research project that would compete with other research projects'.

To help me understand what she means, Evans explains how another research project that was looking into kidney failure, for example, might work. In that project, researchers could test blood, measure urea levels, examine a biopsy, take blood pressure—none of which is available for measuring the success of pain treatments in chronic pain patients. In fact, the *Relieving Pain in America* report specifically addresses this issue: 'In the committee's opinion, current processes within the National Institutes of Health for the review of grants pertaining to pain are suboptimal in that many topics in pain research do not fit within existing study sections, and expertise for the review of submitted proposals is inconsistent.'[36] It makes a series of recommendations to support better assessment of pain research, including designating a lead institute at the National Institutes of Health to move pain research forward, improving processes for the development of novel agents for the control of pain,

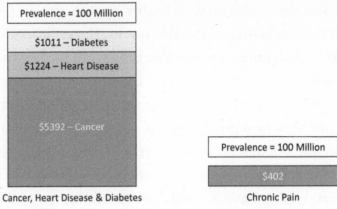

Research spending (in millions) from NIH in 2014 by prevalence
of major diseases
Source: Chronic Pain Research Alliance

expediting the processes for the approval of new pain therapies, encouraging support for interdisciplinary research in pain, and increasing public and private funding for longitudinal research in pain—such as comparative effectiveness research and novel randomised controlled trials—to help ensure patients receive care that works best in both the short and long terms, and to increase the training of pain researchers.

The lack of specific scientific assessment tools and biomarkers for identifying or diagnosing chronic pain make it hard to study. In addition, the ways in which individual patient symptoms vary according to biopsychosocial influences mean treatment efficacy is also hard to study. These complex conditions represent a huge challenge to the research community—but doesn't that make the effort all the more worthwhile? When the AIDS virus broke out in the 1980s, the medical community felt it was impossible to control. Just over thirty years later, AIDS patients are living well and rates of contraction are steadily decreasing. Two patients have even been declared 'cured'.[37]

This is a remarkable achievement of science, and involved a huge effort—not just of tireless campaigners in the LGBTI+ community, but also of governments, industry and research communities backing and supporting the effort. Medicine is capable of great achievements when the will is there.

But chronic pain and, in particular, the chronic overlapping pain conditions, are beset by bad publicity. So many of them, as we've discovered, are contested, the patients disliked by health professionals and significant social stigma attached to them. And pain doesn't actually kill people—it keeps women in the home and out of work, which has no effect on the power structures of society, providing no incentive for action. What research money that has gone into chronic pain conditions has tended not to be involved in understanding the disease mechanism but on psychosomatic aspects: personality types and even body shapes. I wish I was joking.

Not only has the medical research community been disarmingly uninterested in chronic fatigue syndrome, for example—despite it affecting 17 million people worldwide—they have actively suppressed research into it. In 1999, a US Department of Health audit discovered that at least 39 per cent of $23 million the US Congress had allocated to the Center for Disease Control to investigate CFS/ME between 1995 and 1998 had actually been spent on other programs, and that officials provided inaccurate information regarding where the money had gone, Maya Dusenbery reported.[38][39] Even the research that did occur was mainly to look at personality-type profiles of people who get the disease rather than searching for a root cause.

How can we really know if a disease is made up if no one bothers to look into it properly? It wouldn't be the first time a new disease was discovered. But the advent of evidence-based medicine has unwittingly engendered a lack of curiosity in medical practitioners. Dr Lucinda Bateman, a specialist in CFS/ME, told Dusenbery: 'We've taught people that it's not okay to think outside the box. We've implied that if [something] doesn't fit what we know, it's probably not important, or it's probably psychological. It goes in the garbage can. There's no curiosity. That's a very modern change in medicine.'[40]

Dr Kate Young says this type of research is a result of men making knowledge while they look through their own lens at female illness. As an example, she points me to an endometriosis study published in the prestigious *Fertility and Sterility*[41] journal where the researchers assessed women's physical attractiveness by looking at their breast size and their hip width, and then correlated that with the severity of their endo symptoms. She calls it 'insane' they got ethics approval for that research, and while there was a backlash, the researchers defended the work.

But Evans says, 'If you actually look at the young researchers, a lot of them are women, particularly in this area.' In particular, Linda Watkins in the US and Katy Vincent in the UK are making major inroads into understanding female pain. Evans says many young women in science are wanting to follow in their footsteps. 'The biggest problem is with so little support for them in this area, most of them will have to leave research because they won't be able to get a job.'

Is change in the air? A case study of endometriosis
In 2015 when *The Guardian* ran its global investigation into endometriosis, most people had never heard of this disease. It received little media attention, while few governments

(Italy and New Zealand are notable exceptions) paid it any attention in funding or policy. So much has changed since then. In 2018, 'What is endometriosis?' was the question third most frequently asked of Dr Google.[42]

In 2017, the UK's All-Party Parliamentary Group on Women's Health led an investigation into the treatment of women with fibroids and endo. The resulting report found that women in the UK weren't being treated with dignity in the health service, weren't being correctly diagnosed, and weren't given adequate information about their physical, mental and gynaecological health. It also found that the NHS wasn't consistently collecting data—if at all—on endo and fibroids, and that there was no consistent patient pathway for women with these conditions.

Later that year, the National Institute for Health and Care Excellence in England released its first-ever guidance on managing endometriosis. The guidance critically encourages doctors to suspect endo at first presentation in cases of chronic pelvic pain, period pain, deep pain during or after sex, or cyclical gastrointestinal and urinary problems. Speedy referral to gynaecologists is recommended if first-line treatments such as nonsteroidal anti-inflammatory drugs and the combined oral contraceptive pill have no impact after three months. In cases where deep endometriosis involving the bladder, bowel or ureter is suspected or confirmed, women should be referred to specialist endometriosis centres sponsored by the British Society for Gynaecological Endoscopy, which use a multi-disciplinary approach and the latest evidence-based treatments.

Australia has experienced a similar revolution in awareness. In 2017, our minister for health, Greg Hunt, apologised to endometriosis sufferers for the pain they've endured and expressed regret that more hadn't been done to support them. In 2018, his department released a National Action Plan for Endometriosis, developed in conjunction with health-care professionals, patient advocates and researchers. The plan has three key aspects: awareness and education; clinical management and care; and research. It promises to fund awareness-raising campaigns for healthcare professionals, roll out a menstrual education program in schools, develop national clinical guidelines for treatment, reduce the cost burden for patients, and develop surgical accreditation standards so that all endo patients receive quality surgery.

During 2018 and 2019, $15 million in funding was awarded to meet these goals, with $9 million allocated to a contested call for research through Australia's Medical Research Future Fund that leads to non-invasive diagnostic testing, and a better understanding of the causes and underlying disease mechanisms. The University of Adelaide was granted $1.06 million to develop a digital health platform for endometriosis research and support; $2.5 million went to Jean Hailes to establish a clinical research network, as well as additional funding for awareness raising activities among healthcare professionals and a schools program.[43] This is a massive victory for people with endometriosis and a huge credit to the many people, mostly women, who have worked tirelessly for many years to advocate for a better deal for endo patients.

In the United States, policy progress for endo patients has been slower in coming. But public awareness has grown as Lena Dunham has so publicly shared her experiences of the disease. Susan Sarandon, Whoopi Goldberg and Padma Lakshmi, who all have endo, have also contributed to greater awareness of the disease.

The filmmaker Shannon Cohn released a feature-length documentary *Endo What?* in 2016 to raise awareness of endometriosis and to give women facts about it. When the film toured Australia, I talked to Cohn, who told me that she'd made it after realising that in the twenty years since her diagnosis, nothing had changed—not even the delay in diagnosis. She started researching successful social change movements and studied HIV/AIDS campaigns. She realised there were three important lessons: 'One, patients became experts in their disease; two, they organised incredibly well; and three, they weren't afraid to make people in power uncomfortable.'

The US Endo What? campaign reached a milestone in 2018 when it received the support of Democratic Senator Elizabeth Warren and Republican Senator Orrin Hatch for a bipartisan initiative to improve awareness and understanding of endometriosis. Writing for CNN, Hatch shared the profound sadness he felt watching his granddaughter suffer with the disease. 'The widespread prevalence of endometriosis—and the lack of any long-term treatment options—is nothing short of a public health emergency,' he wrote.[44] It resulted in additional funding for endo research from the US Department of Defense. However, policy change, substantial research funding and clinical guidelines haven't yet been forthcoming.

As it did with breast cancer, the speedy and substantial change in awareness of endometriosis has come about from women campaigning for better treatment. Change rarely takes place from within medicine; it happens more frequently because of outside pressure on governments. And governments must make it a priority to fund research and develop guidance for medical treatment so that everyone receives the best available care.

EPILOGUE

We live in an era where distrust in democratic institutions is growing at the same time as trust in pseudoscience and conspiracy theories. In writing this book, I tried to be responsible in unpicking the reasons we find ourselves in a situation where medical science remains so ignorant of women's pain. I've tried to do this carefully in order to lift the burden from the shoulders of individual doctors and nurses. It's not their fault—but they can help fix it.

I believe that medicine urgently needs to have a reckoning. Medical institutions around the world need to look at how they teach women's health in medical school and how they treat women and trans*, intersex and gender non-binary people with complex emotional and physical problems in practice. Medicine needs to be vocal about its past failures and its intent to do better in the future. Governments need to be part of this, to encourage it and to provide the funding for the urgent research required to help women and minorities live better.

Because I have a male doctor as a partner and a nurse as a mother, I have insight into medicine that many don't. I know there are doctors, nurses and many other healthcare practitioners who care and who want to do the right thing by all their patients. I've met and interviewed countless excellent doctors and researchers, both male and female, who are striving to ease everyone's pain and to improve all healthcare experiences.

But many women and minorities don't have this access. There's a palpable anger towards conventional medicine, and doctors in particular, that needs to be confronted. While I was writing this book, I came across a Twitter hashtag, #doctorsaredickheads. This hashtag angered doctors, and I could argue that alienating the people you need to help resolve your problem is counterproductive—but the people who started this hashtag have a right to be angry. A short scroll through their posts reveals a horror story of ignorance, dismissal, prejudice, intolerance and snobbishness by doctors towards their patients with rare or under-researched illnesses.

How is that acceptable?

Doctors need to learn they don't have all the answers, and they need the skills to deal with patients whose symptoms they may not be able to treat very well. They need to listen to, and believe, their patients. As rates of chronic illness continue to grow across the world, this problem won't fix itself. And the longer medicine puts off being part of a conversation, the more people whose trust it loses.

I know a woman who's had so many bad experiences with GPs, she now uses an osteopath as her primary source of medical advice. When forced to go to a GP, she'll only attend an appointment with her male partner, whom she believes GPs listen to more than her. She's a smart, capable woman.

Her experience is an indictment on what should be a healing profession—and it's only one experience.

The number of women and others with female reproductive organs in pain who have gravitated towards the wellness industry is untold. Because I know they come from a well-meaning place, I've chosen not to recount the many fringe treatments recommended to me by caring women. I used to scoff at the wellness industry and its 'ridiculous' claims and 'ridiculous' treatments at 'ridiculous' prices targeted mainly at rich white women. But after four years of researching, talking to women in pain and listening to people's experiences of conventional healthcare and alternative and complementary therapies, I finally understand. I don't blame women for seeking out these views and therapies. They're not stupid, or gullible, or somehow more credulous than others; they're desperate. They're in pain, or they have a symptom that Western medicine can't help with, and they'll try anything for relief. Far from irrational, that's a perfectly reasonable response to being ignored, dismissed or made to feel stupid by a doctor.

When I talked to Dr Kate Young about this phenomenon, she said that most women in her research didn't abandon conventional medicine altogether but added alternative therapy to their healthcare. While some studies have shown a correlation between people who have negative experiences of conventional medicine and the use of alternative healthcare, a study published in the *Journal of the American Medical Association* found that it isn't a predictive factor. That study, however, found that the most frequent health problem treated with alternative therapies was chronic pain (37 per cent), followed by anxiety and chronic fatigue syndrome (31 per cent).[1]

It can't be a coincidence that conventional medicine offers very little relief for these illnesses. Few people would begrudge a person seeking alternative healthcare for symptoms that conventional medicine has no good treatment for.

Young's main issue with alternative therapies is that they often draw upon the same repressive discourses and gender beliefs around women as conventional medicine—such as, because you *can* have a baby, you *should* have a baby, or tracing almost any illness back to the uterus, menstrual cycle or female hormones.

Often people using alternative healthcare don't even think it's that effective, Young says—they just like the fact someone sits down and listens to them. We know that people with doctors who acknowledge their pain and listen to their stories experience less severe pain symptoms, so this idea is hardly revolutionary. It's also harmless.

But what about the alternative therapies that are completely crackpot, cost a lot of money and have the potential to do harm? And why do people continue to seek these out? This is a question medicine needs to ask—and really listen to the answer.

Pain isn't killing us, but it is denying us our full humanity. Refusing to understand this fact of life for women is tearing opportunities from our grasp. And I say, enough!

ACKNOWLEDGEMENTS

To Emily Wilson, who encouraged me to write about endometriosis, and to Katharine Viner, who saw the potential in the story as a global investigation, I owe my heartfelt thanks. And without the EndoActive conference organised by Sylvia Freedman and Lesley Freedman, I would never have had the courage and determination to write about this disease. These are the women who planted the seed in my mind for this book and I will be eternally grateful to them. I couldn't have written this book without the input and knowledge of Dr Babak Adeli and Dr Barbara Cameron, who read every word in early draft form and helped make sure the final manuscript was fair and accurate.

Thank you to Jane Novak, my agent, who believed in this book from the moment I sat in front of her, and to my publisher Kelly Fagan—the support, encouragement and enthusiasm from both of them kept me going. And to my wonderful editors, Kate Goldsworthy and Angela Handley, whose precision and sharp focus have improved the book to no end, and special appreciation to Angela for staying calm when I was really losing my mind while trying to finish the book while working full time (never again!).

It's hard to understate how grateful I am to Dr Susan Evans and Dr Kate Young, who gave me so much of their time, shared so much and helped me take this book in new directions and to greater depth than I could have done without them.

I'm eternally grateful to the other excellent people who spared their time for me: Dr Nikki Stamp, Professor Mark Hutchinson, Dr Clare Fairweather, Dr Anita Saldanha, Emily Nagoski, Dr Rachael Tait, Athena Lamnisos, Mike McRae, Janine Mohamed, Rebecca Manson Jones, Nina Booysen, Tom Rankin and Dr Richard Nguyen. And special thanks to Sharon Williams and her family for allowing me to tell Naomi's story.

I must also give my most heartfelt thanks to the incredible women (and men) who have supported, encouraged and mentored me, and made me a better journalist: Lucy Clark, Emily Wilson, Lenore Taylor and Will Woodward. And to Wendy Harmer and Jane Waterhouse for taking a chance on me when I returned from the wilderness.

I wouldn't be the person I am without my incredible, supportive family: Mum, Dad, Gary, Maggie, Simone, Daniel, Tim, Charlie, Angus, Harry, Matilda, Huntah and all the rest who know I love them. And to my dear friends who've been there through it all, you know who you are. I am forever indebted to you all for your love, support, belief, encouragement and entertainment.

And a final huge hug and thank you to all the women who have felt they could trust me with their stories: this is for all of you.

NOTES

Introduction

1   Gabrielle Jackson, 'I'm not a hypochondriac. I have a disease. All these things that are wrong with me are real, they are endometriosis', *The Guardian*, 28 September 2015, <www.theguardian.com/society/2015/sep/28/im-not-a-hypochondriac-i-have-a-disease-all-these-things-that-are-wrong-with-me-are-real-they-are-endometriosis>.

2   Sarah Boseley, Jessica Glenza and Helen Davidson, 'Endometriosis: The hidden suffering of millions of women revealed', *The Guardian*, 28 September 2015, <www.theguardian.com/society/2015/sep/28/endometriosis-hidden-suffering-millions-women>.

3   '10 leading causes of death in females', *Global Health Observatory*, World Health Organization, 2019, <www.who.int/gho/women_and_health/mortality/situation_trends_causes_death/en>.

4   Ehsan Khan, David Brieger, John Amerena et al., 'Differences in management and outcomes for men and women with ST-elevation myocardial infarction', *Medical Journal of Australia*, 2018, 209(3): 118–23, doi: 10.5694/mja17.01109.

5   C. Noel Bairey Merz, Holly Andersen, Emily Sprague et al., 'Knowledge, attitudes, and beliefs regarding cardiovascular disease in women: The Women's Heart Alliance', *Journal of the American College of Cardiology*, 2017, 70(2): 123–32, doi: 10.1016/j.jacc.2017.05.024.

6   K.K. Hyun, J. Redfern, A. Patel et al., 'Gender inequalities in cardiovascular risk factor assessment and management in primary healthcare', *Heart*, 2017, 103: 492–8, doi: 10.1136/heartjnl-2016-310216.

7   Policy Department Economic and Scientific Policy, *Autoimmune Diseases: Modern diseases,* European Union: Brussels, 2017, <www.europarl.europa.eu/cmsdata/133620/ENVI%202017-09%20WS%20Autoimmune%20diseases%20%20PE%20614.174%20(Publication).pdf>.

8   Caroline Reilly, 'Influx of illness: Will chronic-illness patients get their #MeToo movement?', *Bitch Media*, 6 June 2018, <www.bitchmedia.org/article/chronic-illness-in-literature>.

9   CPPR White Paper, *Impact of Chronic Overlapping Pain Conditions on Public Health and the Urgent Need for Safe and Effective Treatment: 2015 Analysis and Policy Recommendations*, Chronic Pain Research Alliance, May 2015, p. 15, <www.cpralliance.org/public/CPRA_WhitePaper_2015-FINAL-Digital.pdf>.

10 Institute of Medicine (US) Committee on Advancing Pain Research, Care, and Education, *Relieving Pain in America: A blueprint for transforming prevention,*

care, education and research, National Academies Press: Washington, DC, 2011, p. 75, doi: 10.17226/13172.

11 The Eve Appeal, 'It's vitally important to #KnowYourBody', <https://eveappeal.org.uk/news-awareness/know-your-body/>.

12 Toni Hurst, 'The many myths of menopause', Health Central, 11 July 2008, <www.healthcentral.com/article/the-many-myths-of-menopause>.

13 Office of Research on Women's Health, *Report of the National Institutes of Health: Opportunities for research on Women's Health: September 4–6, 1991, Hunt Valley, Maryland*, National Institutes of Health (US), 1992, p. 16, <https://archive.org/stream/reportofnational00nati_2/reportofnational00nati_2_djvu.txt>.

14 Dr Janine Austin Clayton, cited in Roni Caryn Rabin, 'Health researchers will get $10.1 million to counter gender bias in studies', *New York Times*, 23 September 2014, <www.nytimes.com/2014/09/23/health/23gender.html>.

15 Nanette K. Wenger, 'You've come a long way, baby. Cardiovascular health and disease in women: Problems and prospects', *Circulation*, 2004, 109: 558–60, doi: 10.1161/01.CIR.0000117292.19349.D0.

16 Laura Kiesel, 'Women and pain: Disparities in experience and treatment', *Harvard Health Blog*, 9 October 2017, <www.health.harvard.edu/blog/women-and-pain-disparities-in-experience-and-treatment-2017100912562>.

17 Lauren Nicotra, Lisa Loram, Linda Watkins and Mark Hutchinson, 'Toll-like receptors in chronic pain', *Experimental Neurology*, 2012, 234(2): 316–29, doi: 10.1016/j.expneurol.2011.09.038.

18 Esther H. Chen, Frances S. Shofer, Anthony J. Dean et al., 'Gender disparity in analgesic treatment of emergency department patients with acute abdominal pain', *Academic Emergency Medicine*, 2008, 15(5): 414–18, doi: 10.1111/j.1553-2712.2008.00100.x.

19 Diane E. Hoffmann and Anita J. Tarzian, 'The girl who cried pain: A bias against women in the treatment of pain', *Journal of Law, Medicine & Ethics*, 2001, 29: 13–27, doi: 10.2139/ssrn.383803.

20 E.G. Nabel, 'Coronary Heart Disease in women: An ounce of protection', *New England Journal of Medicine*, 2000, 343: 572–4, doi: 10.1056/NEJM200008243430809.

21 L.C. Turtzo and L.D. McCullough, 'Sex differences in stroke', *Cerebrovascular Diseases*, 2008, 26(5): 462–74, doi:10.1159/000155983.

22 Nafees U. Din, Obioha C. Ukoumunne, Greg Rubin et al., 'Age and gender variations in cancer diagnostic intervals in 15 cancers: Analysis of data from the UK Clinical Practice Research Datalink', *PLoS ONE*, 2015, 10(5): e0127717, doi: 10.1371/journal.pone.0127717.

Chapter 1

1 The survey was conducted by PCP Market Research in August 2016 for the Eve Appeal and questioned 1000 women of different ages from across the UK.

2 Olivia Willis, 'A gynaecologist's guide to good vulva and vagina health', ABC, 12 September 2017, <www.abc.net.au/news/health/2017-09-12/a--gynaecologists-guide-to-good-vulva-and-vagina-health/8892230>.

3   M. Simonis, R. Manocha and J.J. Ong, 'Female genital cosmetic surgery: A cross-sectional survey exploring knowledge, attitude and practice of general practitioners', *BMJ Open*, 2016, 6(9): e013010, doi: 10.1136/bmjopen-2016-013010.

4   Lynn Enright, 'Why it matters to call external female genitalia "vulva" not "vagina"', *The Guardian*, 13 February 2019, <www.theguardian.com/commentisfree/2019/feb/12/external-female-genitalia-vulva-vagina-sexual-agency>.

5   Melissa Fyfe, 'Get cliterate: How a Melbourne doctor is redefining female sexuality', *Good Weekend, Sydney Morning Herald*, 8 December 2018, <www.smh.com.au/lifestyle/health-and-wellness/get-cliterate-how-a-melbourne-doctor-is-redefining-female-sexuality-20181203-p50jvv.html>.

6   See <www.allisebastianwolf.com/glitoris!.html>.

7   For more information, see <www.allisebastianwolf.com/glitoris!.html>.

8   John McCann, Sheridan Miyamoto, Cathy Boyle and Kristen Rogers, 'Healing of hymenal injuries in prepubertal and adolescent girls: A descriptive study', *Pediatrics*, May 2007, 119(5): e1094-e1106, doi: 10.1542/peds.2006-0964.

Chapter 2

1   Vibeke Venema, 'The Indian sanitary pad revolution', BBC World Service, 4 March 2014, <www.bbc.com/news/magazine-26260978>.

2   Venema, 'The Indian sanitary pad revolution'.

3   Calla Wahlquist, 'Aboriginal woman in WA fined $500 for stealing $6.75 box of tampons', *The Guardian*, 15 October 2015, <www.theguardian.com/australia-news/2015/oct/15/aboriginal-woman-in-wa-fined-500-for-stealing-675-box-of-tampons>.

4   'Free sanitary products scheme expands in Scotland', *BBC News*, 17 January 2019, <www.bbc.com/news/uk-scotland-46904775>.

5   Sarah Marsh, 'MP breaks House of Commons taboo by discussing her period', *The Guardian*, 29 June 2018, <www.theguardian.com/politics/2018/jun/28/danielle-rowley-breaks-house-of-commons-taboo-discussing-period>.

6   Jane Less, 'Federal election 2016: Labor back-flips on removing GST from tampons', *Sydney Morning Herald*, 9 June 2016, <www.smh.com.au/politics/federal/federal-election-2016-labor-backflips-on-removing-gst-from-tampons-20160608-gpeslb.html>.

7   Nicole Puglise, 'New York lifts "tampon tax"', *The Guardian*, 22 July 2016, <www.theguardian.com/us-news/2016/jul/21/new-york-lifts-tampon-tax>.

8   Kate Young, Jane Fisher and Maggie Kirkman, '"Do mad people get endo or does endo make you mad?": Clinicians' discursive constructions of Medicine and women with endometriosis', *Feminism & Psychology*, 2018, doi:10.1177/0959353518815704.

9   Deirdre Hynds, 'Menstruation is having a moment and it's about bloody time', *Irish Times*, 17 August 2017, <www.irishtimes.com/life-and-style/people/menstruation-is-having-a-moment-and-it-s-about-bloody-time-1.3183679>.

10 Emily Martin, 'The egg and the sperm: How science has constructed a romance based on stereotypical male-female roles', *Signs*, 1991, 16(3): 485–501, <www.jstor.org/stable/3174586?seq=17#page_scan_tab_contents>.

11 Allen J. Wilcox, Clarice R. Weinberg, and Donna D. Baird, 'Timing of sexual intercourse in relation to ovulation', *New England Journal of Medicine*, 1995, 333: 1517–21, <www.nejm.org/doi/full/10.1056/nejm199512073332301>.

12 Kathy K. Niakan, Jinnuo Han, Roger A. Pedersen et al., 'Human pre-implantation embryo development', *Development*, 2012, 139(5): 829–41, doi: 10.1242/dev.060426.

13 Dr Sarah McKay, *The Women's Brain Book: The neuroscience of health, hormones and happiness*, Hachette Australia: Sydney, 2018, p. 92.

14 Nina Brochmann and Ellen Støkken Dahl, *The Wonder Down Under: A user's guide to the vagina*, Yellow Kite: UK, 2018, p. 59.

15 S.E. Romans, D. Kreindler, E. Asllani et al., 'Mood and the menstrual cycle', *Psychotherapy & Psychosomatics*, 2013, 82: 53–60, doi: 10.1159/000339370.

16 Sarah Romans, Rose Clarkson, Gillian Einstein et al., 'Mood and the menstrual cycle: A review of prospective data studies', *Gender Medicine*, 2012, 9(5): 361–84, doi: 10.1016/j.genm.2012.07.003.

17 Jane M. Ussher, *Managing the Monstrous Feminine*, Routledge: UK, 2006, p. 74.

18 David Reuben, *Everything You Always Wanted to Know About Sex* (*But Were Afraid to Ask)*, David McKay and Company: New York, 1969 (1st edn), p. 366.

19 Reuben, *Everything You Always Wanted to Know About Sex**, p. 287.

20 L. Dennerstein, 'Well-being, symptoms and the menopausal transition', *Maturitas*, 1996, 23: 147–57, doi: 10.1016/0378-5122(95)00970-1.

21 R.A. Wilson and T.A. Wilson, 'The fate of the nontreated postmenopausal woman: A plea for the maintenance of adequate estrogen from puberty to the grave', *Journal of the American Geriatrics Society*, 1963, 11: 347–62, doi:10.1111/j.1532-5415.1963.tb00068.x.

22 Richard A. Morton, Jonathan R. Stone and Rama S. Singh, 'Mate choice and the origin of menopause', *PLoS Computational Biology*, 2013, 9(6): e1003092, doi: 10.1371/journal.pcbi.1003092.

23 Morton, Stone and Singh, 'Mate choice and the origin of menopause'.

24 Angela Saini, *Inferior: The true power of women and science that shows it*, Fourth Estate: Great Britain, 2017, p. 228.

25 K.A. Matthews, 'Myths and Realities of the Menopause', *Psychosomatic Medicine*, 1992, 54(1): 1–9, <https://journals.lww.com/psychosomatic medicine/Citation/1992/01000/Myths_and_realities_of_the_ menopause_.1.aspx>.

26 B.N. Ayers, M.J. Forshaw and M.S. Hunter, 'The menopause', *Psychologist*, 2011, 24(5): 348–52.

27 Suzanne Moore, 'Let's see menopausal women on screen—in all their glory', *The Guardian*, 16 March 2018, <www.theguardian.com/commentisfree/2018/ mar/15/menopausal-women-screen-glory-representation-menopause- popular-culture>.

28 Marina Benjamin, 'Don't hide the menopause—celebrate its creative power', *The Guardian*, 29 August 2018, <www.theguardian.com/commentisfree/2018/aug/29/menopause-cafes-women-creative-surge>.

29 Rosemary Leonard, in *Menopause: The answers*, Hachette: UK, 2017, p. 28.

30 Leonard, *Menopause*, p. 97.

31 G. Andrews, W. Hall and M. Teeson, *The Mental Health of Australia*, Commonwealth Department of Aged Care: Canberra, 1999.

32 N. Avis, D. Brambilla, S.M. McKinlay and K. Vass, 'A longitudinal analysis of the association between menopause and depression: Results from the Massachusetts women's health study', *American Journal of Epidemiology*, 1994, 4: 15-21, doi: 10.1016/1047-2797(94)90099-X.

33 Australasian Menopause Society, 'Will menopause affect my sex life?', <www.menopause.org.au/health-info/fact-sheets/will-menopause-affect-my-sex-life>.

34 Ussher, *Managing the Monstrous Feminine*, p. 126.

35 Ussher, *Managing the Monstrous Feminine*, p. 131.

36 American Sociological Association, 'Women more likely than men to initiate divorces, but not non-marital breakups', *ScienceDaily*, 22 August 2015, <www.sciencedaily.com/releases/2015/08/150822154900.htm>.

37 Grace Johnston, *Menopause Essentials: Every woman's guide*, Wilkinson Publishing: Melbourne, 2013, p. 45.

38 Margalit Fox, 'Estelle R. Ramey, 89, who used medical training to rebut sexism, is dead', *New York Times*, 12 September 2006, <www.nytimes.com/2006/09/12/obituaries/12ramey.html>.

39 Carolyn Dean, 'Broken promises: The history of HRT', Hotze, 29 July 2011, <www.hotzehwc.com/2011/07/broken-promises-the-history-of-hrt/>.

40 Writing Group for the Women's Health Initiative Investigators, 'Risks and benefits of estrogen plus progestin in healthy postmenopausal women: Principal results from the Women's Health Initiative Randomized Controlled Trial', *JAMA*, 2002, 288(3): 321–33, doi:10.1001/jama.288.3.321.

41 Million Women Study Collaborators, 'Breast cancer and hormone replacement therapy in the Million Women Study', *The Lancet*, 2003, 362(9382): 419–27, doi: 10.1016/S0140-6736(03)14065-2.

42 T.J. de Villiers, M.L. Gass, D.J. Haines et al., 'Global consensus statement on menopausal hormone therapy', *Climacteric*, 2013, 16(2): 203–4, doi: 10.3109/13697137.2013.771520.

43 US Food and Drug Administration, 'Menopause', <www.fda.gov/consumers/womens-health-topics/menopause>.

44 Australian Menopause Society, 'Bioidentical custom compounded hormone therapy', <www.menopause.org.au/hp/information-sheets/212-bioidentical-hormones-for-menopausal-symptoms>.

45 T.J. de Villiers, J.E. Hall, J.V. Pinkerton et al., 'Revised global consensus statement on menopausal hormone therapy', *Maturitas*, 2016, 91: 153–5, doi: 10.1016/j.maturitas.2016.06.001.

46 Katherine Ellen Foley, 'Five animals experience menopause. Four of them

live underwater', *Quartz*, 30 August 2018, <https://qz.com/1372767/twice-as-many-animals-go-through-menopause-as-scientists-previously-thought/>.

47 Pat Lee Shipman, 'Why is human childbirth so painful?', *American Scientist*, 2013, 101(6): 426, <www.americanscientist.org/article/why-is-human-childbirth-so-painful>, doi: 10.1511/2013.105.426.

48 Simone de Beauvoir, *The Second Sex*, Vintage Books: London, trans. Constance Borde and Sheila Malovany-Chevallier, 2009 [1949], p. 66.

49 Grace Johnston, *Menopause Essentials: every woman's guide*, Wilkinson Publishing: Melbourne, 2013, p. 10.

50 Rose George, '"It feels impossible to beat": How I was floored by menopause', *The Guardian*, 16 August 2018, <www.theguardian.com/news/2018/aug/16/it-feels-impossible-to-beat-how-i-was-floored-by-menopause>.

51 R. Bauld and R.F. Brown, 'Stress, psychological distress, psychosocial factors, menopause symptoms and physical health in women', *Maturitas*. 2009, 62(2): 160–5, doi: 10.1016/j.maturitas.2008.12.004.

52 Ussher, *Managing the Monstrous Feminine*, p. 145.

53 Marina Benjamin, 'Don't hide the menopause—celebrate its creative power', *The Guardian*, 29 August 2018, <www.theguardian.com/commentisfree/2018/aug/29/menopause-cafes-women-creative-surge>.

54 Betty Friedan, *The Fountain of Age*, Simon & Schuster Paperbacks: New York, 2006 [1993], p. 158.

Chapter 3

1 Trina Jones, cited in Ritu Prasad, 'Serena Williams and the trope of the "angry black woman"', BBC News, 11 September 2018, <www.bbc.com/news/world-us-canada-45476500>.

2 '"One must respect the game": French Open says "non" to Serena's catsuit', *The Guardian*, 25 August 2018, <www.theguardian.com/sport/2018/aug/24/serena-catsuit-french-open-dress-code>.

3 *Q&A*, ABC TV, 12 July 2016; Van Badham, 'I'm still reeling from Q&A—but not because I was called "hysterical"', 12 July 2016, <www.theguardian.com/commentisfree/2016/jul/12/im-still-reeling-from-qa-but-not-because-i-was-called-hysterical>.

4 Mike McRae, *Unwell: What makes a disease a disease?*, UQP: Brisbane, 2018, p. 20.

5 George Rousseau, 'A "strange pathology": Hysteria in the early modern world, 1500–1800', in Sander L. Gilman, Helen King, Roy Porter, G.S. Rousseau and Elaine Showalter, *Hysteria Beyond Freud*, University of California Press: Berkeley and Los Angeles, CA, 1993, p. 92.

6 Helen King, *Hippocrates' Woman: Reading the female body in Ancient Greece*, Taylor & Francis: US, 1998.

7 Andrew Scull, *Hysteria: The disturbing history*, Oxford University Press: UK, 2009, p. 12.

8 McRae, *Unwell*, p. 20.
9 Helen King, 'Once upon a text: Hysteria from Hippocrates', in *Hysteria Beyond Freud*, p. 15.
10 Robert R. Turner and Charles Edgley, 'From witchcraft to drugcraft: Biochemistry as mythology', *Social Science Journal*, 1983, 20:1.
11 Scull, *Hysteria*, p. 20.
12 Scull, *Hysteria*, p. 21.
13 Rousseau, in *Hysteria Beyond Freud*, p. 93.
14 Rousseau, in *Hysteria Beyond Freud*, p. 137.
15 Rousseau, in *Hysteria Beyond Freud*, p. 94.
16 Rousseau, in *Hysteria Beyond Freud*, p. 157.
17 Rousseau, in *Hysteria Beyond Freud*, p. 158.
18 King, in *Hysteria Beyond Freud*, p. 13.
19 Scull, *Hysteria*, p. 58.
20 Barbara Ehrenreich and Deirdre English, *Complaints and Disorders: The sexual politics of sickness*, The Feminist Press: New York, 2011 [1973], p. 36.
21 Scull, *Hysteria*, p. 64.
22 Elaine Showalter, 'Hysteria, feminism and gender', in *Hysteria Beyond Freud*, p. 301.
23 Showalter, in *Hysteria Beyond Freud*, pp. 302–3.
24 Charlotte Perkins Gilman, *The Man-Made World: Our androcentric culture*, The Floating Press: Auckland, 2011 [1911], p. 32.
25 Cited in Scull, *Hysteria*, pp. 65–6.
26 Robert Brudenell Carter, *On the Pathology and Treatment of Hysteria*, J. Churchill: London, 1853, p. 55.
27 Brudenell Carter, *On the Pathology and Treatment of Hysteria*, p. 69.
28 Brudenell Carter, *On the Pathology and Treatment of Hysteria*, p. 112.
29 Carroll Smith-Rosenberg and Charles Rosenberg, 'The female animal: Medical and biological views of woman and her role in nineteenth century America', *Journal of American History*, 1973, 60(2): 332–56, doi: 10.2307/2936779.
30 Scull, *Hysteria*, p. 72.
31 Ehrenreich and English, *Complaints and Disorders*, p. 59.
32 Scull, *Hysteria*, p. 77.
33 McRae, *Unwell*, p. 144.
34 Isaac Baker Brown, *On the Curability of Certain Forms of Insanity, Epilepsy, Catalepsy, and Hysteria in Females*, Robert Hardwicke: London, 1866.
35 Francis Seymour Haden, cited in 'The Debate at the Obstetrical Society', *British Medical Journal*, 6 April 1867, p. 396.
36 Scull, *Hysteria*, p. 88.
37 A.M. Hamilton, 'The abuse of oophorectomy in diseases of the nervous system', *New York Medical Journal*, 1893, 57: 181.
38 R.T. Edes, 'Points in the diagnosis and treatment of some obscure neuroses', *Journal of the American Medical Association*, 1896, 27: 1080.

39 Howard A. Kelly, 'Conservatism in ovariotomy', *Journal of the American Medical Association*, 1896, 26: 251.

40 George Beard, *American Nervousness*, Putman: New York, 1881, p. 17.

41 Showalter, in *Hysteria Beyond Freud*, p. 297.

42 Showalter, in *Hysteria Beyond Freud*, p. 297.

43 Ussher, *The Madness of Women*, p. 9.

44 Showalter, in *Hysteria Beyond Freud*, p. 297.

45 Scull, *Hysteria*, p. 107.

46 Rousseau, in *Hysteria Beyond Freud*, p. 185.

47 Showalter, in *Hysteria Beyond Freud*, pp. 307–8.

48 Cited in Scull, *Hysteria*, pp. 120–1.

49 Showalter, in *Hysteria Beyond Freud*, p. 123.

50 Mark S. Micale, 'Hysteria and its historiography: A review of past and present writings, II,' *History of Science*, 1989, 27(4): 319–51, doi: 10.1177/007327538902700401.

51 Scull, *Hysteria*, p. 134.

52 Scull, *Hysteria*, pp. 135–6.

53 Scull, *Hysteria*, p. 135.

54 Showalter, in *Hysteria Beyond Freud*, p. 316.

55 Scull, *Hysteria*, p. 145.

56 Showalter, in *Hysteria Beyond Freud*, p. 317.

57 Showalter, in *Hysteria Beyond Freud*, p. 317.

58 Quoted in Scull, *Hysteria*, p. 150.

59 Scull, *Hysteria*, p. 159.

60 King, in *Hysteria Beyond Freud*, pp. 9–10.

61 Rousseau, in *Hysteria Beyond Freud*, p. 186.

62 Sally Rooney, *Conversations with Friends*, Faber & Faber: London, 2017, p. 124.

Chapter 4

1 Young, Fisher and Kirkman, 'Do mad people get endo or does endo make you mad?'

2 Ehrenreich and English, *Complaints and Disorders*, pp. 31–8

3 Kate Manne, *Down Girl: The logic of misogyny*, Penguin Random House: UK, 2019, p. xiii.

4 Rebecca Solnit, 'The fall of Harvey Weinstein should be a moment to challenge extreme masculinity', *The Guardian*, 12 October 2017, <www.theguardian.com/commentisfree/2017/oct/12/challenge-extreme-masculinity-harvey-weinstein-degrading-women>.

5 Afua Hirsch, *Brit(ish): On race, identity and belonging*, Jonathan Cape: London, 2018, p. 114.

6 Patricia Park, 'The Madame Butterfly Effect: Tracing the History of a Fetish', *Bitch Media*, 30 July 2014, <www.bitchmedia.org/article/the-madame-butterfly-effect-asian-fetish-history-pop-culture>.

7   Statistic on Violence Against API Women, Asian Pacific Institute on Gender-Based Violence, <www.api-gbv.org/about-gbv/statistics-violence-against-api-women/>.

8   Manne, *Down Girl*, p. 300.

9   Manne, *Down Girl*, p. 301.

10 Ussher, *The Madness of Women*, p. 31.

11 Ussher, *The Madness of Women*, p. 32.

12 Emily Nagoski, *Come as You Are: The surprising new science that will transform your sex life*, Simon & Schuster: New York, 2015, p. 2.

13 Lili Loofbourow, 'The female price of male pleasure', *The Week*, 25 January 2018, <https://theweek.com/articles/749978/female-price-male-pleasure>.

14 Loofbourow, 'The female price of male pleasure'.

15 Loofbourow, 'The female price of male pleasure'.

16 OMGYes, <www.omgyes.com/>.

17 Nagoski, *Come as You Are*, p. 43.

18 Nagoski, *Come as You Are*, p. 69.

19 Aziz Ansari with Eric Klinenberg, *Modern Romance: An investigation*, Penguin: New York, 2015.

20 Steven Pinker, 'Boys will be boys: An evolutionary explanation for Presidents behaving badly', *New Yorker*, 9 February 1998, pp. 30–1.

21 Jethro Mullen and Masoud Popalzai, 'Woman stoned to death in Afghanistan over accusation of adultery', CNN, 4 November 2015, <https://edition.cnn.com/2015/11/04/asia/afghanistan-taliban-woman-stoning/index.html>.

22 'Female genital mutilation: Prevalence of FGM', World Health Organization, <www.who.int/reproductivehealth/topics/fgm/prevalence/en/>.

23 McRae, *Unwell*, p. 142.

24 'Esther Perel Interview on Sex, Power and Control', *Speaking of Sex with the Pleasure Mechanics*, 15 December 2017, <https://podtail.com/en/podcast/speaking-of-sex-with-the-pleasure-mechanics/esther-perel-interview-on-sex-power-and-desire/>.

25 'Facts and figures: Ending violence against women', UN Women, <www.unwomen.org/en/what-we-do/ending-violence-against-women/facts-and-figures>.

26 'Facts and figures: Ending violence against women', UN Women.

27 'World Report on Violence and Health', World Health Organization 2002, p. 89, <www.who.int/violence_injury_prevention/violence/world_report/en/>.

28 'Facts and figures: Ending violence against women', UN Women.

29 'Victims of Sexual Violence: Statistics', Rainn, <www.rainn.org/statistics/victims-sexual-violence>.

30 'Social, economic and legal empowerment of Egyptian women', United Nations, 26 November 2013, p. 5, <www.undp.org/content/dam/egypt/docs/Women%20Empowerment/Women_Empowerment_Swedish_Proposal_26Nov2013%20(2).pdf>.

31 'Sexual assault and the LGBTQ Community', Human Rights Campaign, <www.hrc.org/resources/sexual-assault-and-the-lgbt-community>.

32 'Family, domestic and sexual violence in Australia, 2018', Australian Institute of Health and Welfare, 28 February 2018, <www.aihw.gov.au/reports/domestic-violence/family-domestic-sexual-violence-in-australia-2018/contents/summary>.

33 Hannana Siddiqui, 'Counting the cost: BME women and gender-based violence in the UK', *IPPR Progressive Review*, 2018, 24(4): 361–8, <https://onlinelibrary.wiley.com/doi/full/10.1111/newe.12076>.

34 Ussher, *The Madness of Women*, p. 112.

35 Esther Perel Interview on Sex, Power and Control', *Speaking of Sex with the Pleasure Mechanics*.

36 Anne Summers, *Damned Whores and God's Police*, Penguin: Ringwood, 1975.

37 'Trends in the prevalence of sexual behaviors and HIV testing', *National Youth Risk Behavior Survey: 1991–2015*, US Center for Disease Control, <www.cdc.gov/healthyyouth/data/yrbs/pdf/trends/2015_us_sexual_trend_yrbs.pdf>.

38 Cicely Marston, 'All too often, anal sex isn't about young women's desires', *The Conversation*, 14 August 2014.

39 World Health Organization (WHO), *Defining Sexual Health*, Department of Reproductive Health and Research, WHO: Geneva, 2006, p. 5, <www.who.int/reproductivehealth/publications/sexual_health/defining_sexual_health.pdf?ua=1>.

40 United Nations Population Fund, *Unfinished Business: The pursuit of rights and choices for all, State of World Population 2019*, UNFPA: New York, 2019 <www.unfpa.org/sites/default/files/pub-pdf/UNFPA_PUB_2019_EN_State_of_World_Population.pdf>.

41 'Esther Perel Interview on Sex, Power and Control', *Speaking of Sex with the Pleasure Mechanics*.

42 Barbara Ehrenreich and Deirdre English, *Complaints and Disorders: The sexual politics of sickness*, 2011 (2nd edn), The Feminist Press: New York, pp. 50–1.

43 Ehrenreich and Deirdre English, *Complaints and Disorders*, p. 57.

44 K. Young, J. Fisher and M. Kirkman, 'Endometriosis and fertility: Women's accounts of healthcare', *Human Reproduction*, 2016, 31(3): 554–62, doi: 10.1093/humrep/dev337.

45 Young, Fisher and Kirkman, 'Endometriosis and fertility'.

46 Karin Hammarberg, Veronica Collins, Carol Holden et al., 'Men's knowledge, attitudes and behaviours relating to fertility', *Human Reproduction Update*, 2017 23(4): 458–80, doi: 10.1093/humupd/dmx005.

47 Ian Sample, 'Men are affected by the biological clock as well, researchers find', *The Guardian*, 3 July 2017, <www.theguardian.com/science/2017/jul/02/men-are-affected-by-the-biological-clock-as-well-researchers-find>.

48 Ian Sample, 'Scientists warn that biological clock affects male fertility', *The Guardian*, 7 July 2008, <www.theguardian.com/society/2008/jul/07/health.children>.

49 B.M. D'Onofrio, M.E. Rickert, E. Frans et al., 'Paternal age at childbearing and offspring psychiatric and academic morbidity', *JAMA Psychiatry*, 2014, 71(4): 432–8, doi:10.1001/jamapsychiatry.2013.4525.

50 Geeta Nargund, 'Men, we need to talk about sperm', *The Guardian*, 23 June 2017, <www.theguardian.com/commentisfree/2017/jun/23/men-we-need-to-talk-about-sperm-biological-clocks>.

51 Melissa Davey, 'Johnson & Johnson withdraws pelvic mesh device from Australian market', *The Guardian*, 23 January 2018, <www.theguardian.com/society/2018/jan/23/johnson-johnson-withdraws-pelvic-vaginal-mesh-device-from-australian-market>.

52 Hannah Devlin, '"Scandal" of vaginal mesh removal rates revealed by NHS records', *The Guardian*, 16 August 2017, <www.theguardian.com/society/2017/aug/15/scandal-of-vaginal-mesh-removal-rates-revealed-by-nhs-records>.

53 D. Herbenick, V. Schick, S.A. Sanders et al., 'Pain experienced during vaginal and anal intercourse with other-sex partners: Findings from a nationally representative probability study in the United States', *Journal of Sexual Medicine*, 12(4): 1040–51, doi: 10.1111/jsm.12841.

54 Susan Berger, 'Vaginal mesh has caused health problems in many women, even as some surgeons vouch for its safety and efficacy', *The Washington Post*, 20 January 2019, <www.washingtonpost.com/national/health-science/vaginal-mesh-has-caused-health-problems-in-many-women-even-as-some-surgeons-vouch-for-its-safety-and-efficacy/2019/01/18/1c4a23-32-ff0f-11e8-ad40-cdfd0e0dd65a_story.html?utm_term=.9ca46341708e>.

55 Christopher Knaus, 'Pelvic mesh victims disgusted at suggestion of anal sex as solution', *The Guardian*, 28 August 2017, <www.theguardian.com/australia-news/2017/aug/28/pelvic-mesh-victims-disgusted-at-suggestion-of-sodomy-as-solution>.

Chapter 5

1 Ussher, *The Madness of Women*, p. 124.

2 'Our stories: The women mutilated by Emil Gayed', *The Guardian*, 7 February 2019, <www.theguardian.com/australia-news/ng-interactive/2019/feb/07/our-stories-the-women-mutilated-by-emil-gayed>.

3 Saini, *Inferior*, p. 42.

4 A. Tsang, M. Von Korff, S. Lee et al., 'Common chronic pain conditions in developed and developing countries: gender and age differences and comorbidity with depression-anxiety disorder', *Journal of Pain: Official journal of the American Pain Society*, 2008, 9(10): 883–91, doi: 10.1016/j.jpain.2008.05.005.

5 Maya Dusenbery, *Doing Harm: The truth about how bad medicine and lazy*

science leave women dismissed, misdiagnosed, and sick, HarperCollins: New York, 2018, p. 20.

6   Melissa Davey, 'Birth control pills should be available over the counter, advocates say', 23 October 2018, <www.theguardian.com/ australia-news/2018/oct/22/birth-control-pills-should-be-available-over-the-counter-advocates-say>.

7   Young, Fisher and Kirkman, 'Do mad people get endo or does endo make you mad?'.

8   Young, Fisher and Kirkman, 'Do mad people get endo or does endo make you mad?', pp. 1, 7.

9   Young, Fisher and Kirkman, 'Do mad people get endo or does endo make you mad?'.

10 Young, Fisher and Kirkman, 'Do mad people get endo or does endo make you mad?'.

11 Young, Fisher and Kirkman, 'Endometriosis and fertility'.

12 K. Young, M. Kirkman, S. Holton et al., 'Fertility experiences in women reporting endometriosis: Findings from the Understanding Fertility Management in Contemporary Australia survey', *The European Journal of Contraception & Reproductive Healthcare*, 2018, 23(6): 434–40, doi: 10.1080/13625187.2018.1539163.

13 Sylvia Freedman, 'With endometriosis, shouldn't "let's get you well" come before "let's get you pregnant"?', *The Guardian*, 19 February 2016, <www. theguardian.com/commentisfree/2016/feb/19/with-endometriosis-shouldnt-lets-get-you-well-come-before-lets-get-you-pregnant>.

14 Judith H. Lichtman, Erica C. Leifheit-Limson, Emi Watanabe et al., 'Symptom recognition and healthcare experiences of young women with acute myocardial infarction', *Circulation*, 2015, 8: S31–S38, doi: 10.1161/ CIRCOUTCOMES.114.001612.

15 Manne, *Down Girl*, p. xix.

16 J. Strong, T. Mathews, R. Sussex et al., 'Pain language and gender differences when describing a past pain event', *Pain*, 2009, 145(1–2): 86–95, doi: 10.1016/j.pain.2009.05.018.

17 Gabrielle R. Chiaramonte and Ronald Friend, 'Medical students' and residents' gender bias in the diagnosis, treatment, and interpretation of coronary heart disease symptoms', *Health Psychology*, 2006, 25(3): 255–66, doi: 10.1037/0278-6133.25.3.255.

18 'Medical sexism: Women's heart disease symptoms often dismissed', ABC7 Los Angeles, <https://abc7.com/archive/8416664/>.

19 N. Fnais, C. Soobiah, M.H. Chen et al., 'Harassment and discrimination in medical training: A systematic review and meta-analysis', *Academic Medicine*, 2014, 89(5): 817–27, doi: 10.1097/ACM.0000000000000200.

20 Pauline Anderson, 'Doctors' suicide rate highest of any profession', WebMD, 8 May 2018, <www.webmd.com/mental-health/news/20180508/doctors-suicide-rate-highest-of-any-profession#1>.

21 B.B. Arnetz, L.G. Hörte, A. Hedberg et al., 'Suicide patterns among physicians related to other academics as well as to the general population", *Acta Psychiatrica Scandinavica*. 1987, 75(2): 139–43, doi: 10.1111/j.1600-0447.1987.tb02765.x.

22 Allison J. Milner, Humaira Maheen, Marie M. Bismark and Matthew J. Spittal, 'Suicide by health professionals: A retrospective mortality study in Australia, 2001–2012', *Medical Journal of Australia*, 2016, 205(6): 260–5, doi: 10.5694/mja15.01044.

23 'Sexual harassment rife in medical profession, warns surgeon', *AM*, ABC Radio, 7 March 2015, <www.abc.net.au/am/content/2015/s4193059.htm>.

24 Louise Stone, Kirsty Douglas and Christine Phillips, 'Beyond zero tolerance: Sexual abuse in medicine', *MJA InSight*, 18 June 2018, <https://insightplus.mja.com.au/2018/23/beyond-zero-tolerance-sexual-abuse-in-medicine/>.

25 Stone, Douglas and Phillips, 'Beyond zero tolerance: Sexual abuse in medicine'.

26 Ranjana Srivastava, 'How doctors treat doctors may be medicine's secret shame', *The Guardian*, 6 February 2015, <www.theguardian.com/commentisfree/2015/feb/06/how-doctors-treat-doctors-may-be-medicines-secret-shame>.

27 Georgina Dent, 'Medical training is a tragedy waiting to happen', *The Guardian*, 16 May 2017, <www.theguardian.com/commentisfree/2017/may/16/medical-training-is-a-tragedy-waiting-to-happen-we-shouldnt-be-silent-about-it>.

28 'Urgent action needed to improve the mental health and save the lives of Australian doctors and medical students', Beyond Blue, 7 October 2013, <www.beyondblue.org.au/media/media-releases/media-releases/action-to-improve-the-mental-health-of-australian-doctors-and-medical-students>.

29 '2016 medical students statistics', 2016, Medical Deans Australia and New Zealand, <www.medicaldeans.org.au/>.

30 M.M. Walton, 'Sexual equality, discrimination and harassment in medicine: It's time to act', *Medical Journal of Australia*, 2015, 203(4): 167–9, doi: 10.5694/mja15.00379.

31 T.C. Cheng, A. Scott, S.H. Jeon et al., 'What factors influence the earnings of general practitioners and medical specialists? Evidence from the medicine in Australia: Balancing employment and life survey', *Health Economics*, 2012, 21(11): 1300–17, doi: 10.1002/hec.1791.

32 Abi Rimmer, 'Male GPs earn 33% more than female GPs, finds pay review', *BMJ*, 2019, 364, doi: 10.1136/bmj.l1510.

33 Parija Kavilanz, 'The gender pay gap for women doctors is big—and getting worse', CNN Business, 14 March 2018, <https://money.cnn.com/2018/03/14/news/economy/gender-pay-gap-doctors/index.html>.

34 Nicole Seebacher, 'Gender equity in medical specialities', Level Medicine,

<http://levelmedicine.org.au/resources/completed-fellowship-papers/gender-equity-in-medical-specialties/>.

35 Brad N. Greenwood, Seth Carnahan and Laura Huang, 'Patient–physician gender concordance and increased mortality among female heart attack patients', *PNAS*, 2018, 115(34): 8569–74, doi: 10.1073/pnas.1800097115.

36 J. Howick, L. Steinkopf, A. Ulyte et al., 'How empathetic is your healthcare practitioner? A systematic review and meta-analysis of patient surveys', *BMC Medical Education*, 2017, 17: 136, doi: 10.1186/s12909-017-0967-3.

37 Yusuke Tsugawa, Anupam B. Jena, Jose F. Figueroa et al., 'Physician gender and outcomes of hospitalized medicare beneficiaries in the U.S.', *JAMA Internal Medicine*, 19 December 2016, doi: 10.1001/jamainternmed.2016.7875.

38 Helen Dickinson and Marie Bismark, 'Female doctors in Australia are hitting glass ceilings—why?', *The Conversation*, 6 January 2016, <https://theconversation.com/female-doctors-in-australia-are-hitting-glass-ceilings-why-51325>.

39 Anonymous GP, 'Female GPs wouldn't have to charge more if Medicare paid properly', *The Guardian*, 24 May 2018, <www.theguardian.com/commentisfree/2018/may/24/female-gps-wouldnt-have-to-charge-more-if-medicare-paid-properly>.

40 Casey Johnston, 'If men had to get IUDs, they'd get epidurals and a hospital stay', *The Outline*, 2 October 2018, <https://theoutline.com/post/6323/if-men-had-to-get-iuds-theyd-get-epidurals-and-a-hospital-stay?zd=1&zi=z5weupuh>.

41 Korin Miller, 'IUD insertions are up 10 percent since the election', *Self*, 26 January 2017, <www.self.com/story/iud-insertions-election-spike>.

42 Cinnamon Janzer, 'Are doctors underestimating the pain of IUD insertion?', *Self*, 6 October 2017, <www.self.com/story/are-doctors-underestimating-the-pain-of-iud-insertion>.

43 Rebecca O'Hara, Heather Rowe, Louise Roufeil and Jane Fisher, 'Should endometriosis be managed within a chronic disease framework? An analysis of national policy documents', *Australian Health Review*, 2018, 42, 627–34, doi: 10.1071/AH17185.

44 Jason Abbott, 'Multiple surgeries aren't the best care for endometriosis. Ask Lena Dunham,' *The Guardian*, 19 February 2018, <www.theguardian.com/commentisfree/2018/feb/19/multiple-surgeries-arent-the-best-care-for-endometriosis-ask-lena-dunham>.

45 Pelvic Pain Steering Committee, *The $6 Billion Woman and the $600 Million Girl: The pelvic pain report*, 2011, p. 50, <http://fpm.anzca.edu.au/documents/pelvic_pain_report_rfs.pdf>.

46 Young, Fisher and Kirkman, 'Do mad people get endo or does endo make you mad?', p. 10.

47 M.C. Howell, 'What medical schools teach about women', *New England Journal of Medicine*, 1974, 291(13): 304–7.

48 Dusenbery, *Doing Harm*, p. 12.

49 Susan Sontag, *Illness as Metaphor and AIDS and Its Metaphors*, Picador: New York, 1990 [*Illness*: 1978, *AIDS*: 1989], p. 55.

50 Young, Fisher and Kirkman, 'Do mad people get endo or does endo make you mad?', p. 6.

51 Susan F. Evans, Tiffany A. Brooks, Adrian J. Esterman et al., 'The comorbidities of dysmenorrhea: A clinical survey comparing symptom profile in women with and without endometriosis', *Journal of Pain Research*, 2018, 11: 3181–94, doi: 10.2147/JPR.S179409.

52 APPG, *Informed Choice? Giving women control of their healthcare*, All-Party Parliamentary Group on Women's Health, p. 21, <https://static1.squarespace.com/static/5757c9a92eeb8124fc5b9077/t/58d8c98b1b10e366b431ba06/1490602405791/APPG+Womens+Health+March+2017+web+title.pdf>.

53 *Informed Choice? Giving women control of their healthcare*, All-Party Parliamentary Group on Women's Health, pp. 21–2.

54 Young, Fisher and Kirkman, 'Do mad people get endo or does endo make you mad?'

55 Roter, cited in Jerome Groopman, *How Doctors Think*, Scribe: Melbourne, 2007, p. 18.

56 Michael Bliss, 'William Osler: A life in medicine', *BMJ*, 2000, 321: 1087, doi: 10.1136/bmj.321.7268.1087/a.

57 Jagdeep Singh Gandhi, 'Re: William Osler: A life in medicine', *BMJ*, 15 July 2014, <www.bmj.com/content/321/7268/1087.2/rr/760724>.

58 Dusenbery, *Doing Harm*, p. 105.

59 Martin A. Makary and Michael Daniel, 'Medical error—the third leading cause of death in the US', *BMJ*, 2016, 353: i2139, doi: 10.1136/bmj.i2139.

60 Groopman, *How Doctors Think*, pp. 69–72.

61 Melissa Davey, 'Death of Indigenous woman turned away from NSW hospital "preventable"', 14 July 2016, <www.theguardian.com/australia-news/2016/jul/14/death-of-pregnant-indigenous-woman-preventable-says-mother>.

62 AIHW, 'Deaths in Australia', Australian Institute of Health and Welfare, 18 July 2018, <www.aihw.gov.au/reports/life-expectancy-death/deaths/contents/life-expectancy>.

63 In 2012–2014 the MMR for Aboriginal and Torres Strait Islander women was 2.4 times that of other Australian women: 13.3 per 100,000 women giving birth versus 5.6 per 100,000 women giving birth: AIHW, 'Maternal deaths in Australia 2012–2014', Australian Institute of Health and Welfare, 8 December 2017, <www.aihw.gov.au/reports/mothers-babies/maternal-deaths-in-australia-2012-2014/contents/risk-factors-for-maternal-death>.

64 Melissa Davey, 'Death of Indigenous woman turned away from NSW hospital "preventable"'.

65 Author's notes from the inquest.

66 A. Singhal, Y.-Y. Tien and R.Y. Hsia, 'Racial-ethnic disparities in opioid prescriptions at emergency department visits for conditions commonly

associated with prescription drug abuse, *PLoS ONE*, 2016, 11(8): e0159224, doi: 10.1371/journal.pone.0159224.

67 Kelly M. Hoffman, Sophie Trawalter, Jordan R. Axt and M. Norman Oliver, 'Racial bias in pain assessment and treatment recommendations, and false beliefs about biological differences between blacks and whites', *PNAS*, 2016, 113(16): 4296–301, doi: 10.1073/pnas.1516047113.

68 Keisha Ray, cited in Amanda Holpuch, 'Black patients half as likely to receive pain medication as white patients', study finds', *The Guardian*, 11 August 2016, <www.theguardian.com/science/2016/aug/10/black-patients-bias-prescriptions-pain-management-medicine-opioids>.

Chapter 6

1   IASP, 'IASP terminology', International Association for the Study of Pain, <www.iasp-pain.org/Education/Content.aspx?ItemNumber=1698#Pain>.

2   Institute of Medicine (US) Committee on Advancing Pain Research, Care, and Education, *Relieving Pain in America*, pp. 31–2.

3   Michael J. Cousin and Rollin M. Gallagher, *Fast Facts: Chronic and cancer pain*, 2017 (4th edn), Health Press: UK, p. 5.

4   Institute of Medicine (US) Committee on Advancing Pain Research, Care, and Education, *Relieving Pain in America*, p. 32.

5   Kristina Fiore, 'Is pain a public health crisis?' Medpage Today, 4 April 2015, <www.medpagetoday.com/painmanagement/painmanagement/50826>.

6   Institute of Medicine (US) Committee on Advancing Pain Research, Care, and Education, *Relieving Pain in America*, p. 1.

7   J.D. Greenspan, R.M. Craft, L. LeResche et al., 'Studying sex and gender differences in pain and analgesia: A consensus report', *Pain*, 2007, 132 (Suppl. 1): S26–S45, doi: 10.1016/j.pain.2007.10.014.

8   Christel Perquin, Alice Hazebroek-Kampschreur, Joke Hunfeld et al., 'Pain in children and adolescents: A common experience', *Pain*, 2000, 87(1): pp. 51–8, doi: 10.1016/S0304-3959(00)00269-4.

9   John Steege and Matthew Siedhoff, 'Chronic pelvic pain', *Obstetrics & Gynecology*, 2014, 124(3): 616–29, doi: 10.1097/AOG.0000000000000417.

10 C.P. Lobo, A.R. Pfalzgraf, V. Giannetti and G. Kanyongo, 'Impact of invalidation and trust in physicians on health outcomes in fibromyalgia patients', *The Primary Care Companion for CNS Disorders*, 2014, 16(5), doi: 10.4088/PCC.14m01664.

11 Lydia Coxon, Andrew W. Horne and Katy Vincent, 'Pathophysiology of endometriosis-associated pain: A review of pelvic and central nervous system mechanisms', *Best Practice & Research Clinical Obstetrics and Gynaecology*, 2018, 51: 53–67, doi: 10.1016/j.bpobgyn.2018.01.014.

12 Kiesel, 'Women and pain'.

13 Dusenbery, *Doing Harm*, p. 180.

14 IASP, 'Pain in Women', International Association for the Study of Pain, <www.iasp-pain.org/GlobalYear/PaininWomen>.

15 Hoffmann and Tarzian, 'The girl who cried pain'.

16 P.A. Johnson, L. Goldman, E.J. Orav et al., 'Gender differences in the management of acute chest pain: Support for the "Yentl syndrome"', *Journal of General Internal Medicine*, 1996, 11(4): 209–17.

17 Hoffmann and Tarzian, 'The girl who cried pain'.

18 Hoffmann and Tarzian, 'The girl who cried pain'.

19 Bendelow, cited in Hoffmann and Tarzian, 'The girl who cried pain'.

20 Hoffmann and Tarzian, 'The girl who cried pain'.

21 IASP, 'Pain in Women'.

22 Victoria M. Grace, 'Problems of communication, diagnosis, and treatment experienced by women using the New Zealand health services for chronic pelvic pain: A quantitative analysis', *Health Care for Women International*, 1995, 16(6): 521–35, doi: 10.1080/07399339509516207.

23 Pelvic Pain Steering Committee, *The $6 Billion Woman and the $600 Million Girl: The pelvic pain report*, p. 8.

24 IASP, 'Chronic pelvic pain', Fact Sheet, Global Year Against Pain in Women, International Association for the Study of Pain, 2007, <www.iasp-pain.org/Advocacy/Content.aspx?ItemNumber=1107>.

25 Caroline Reilly, 'The senseless ubiquity of pain in women', Rewire News, 23 November 2018, <https://rewire.news/article/2018/11/23/the-senseless-ubiquity-of-women-in-pain/>.

26 Ellie Harrison, 'Women are born with pain built in—Kristin Scott Thomas's epic speech on *Fleabag*', *Radio Times*, 19 March 2019, <www.radiotimes.com/news/tv/2019-03-19/women-are-born-with-pain-built-in-kristin-scott-thomass-epic-speech-on-fleabag/>.

27 Pelvic Pain Steering Committee, *The $6 Billion Woman and the $600 Million Girl: The pelvic pain report*, p. 8.

28 Steege and Siedhoff, 'Chronic pelvic pain'.

29 Pelvic Pain Steering Committee, *The $6 Billion Woman and the $600 Million Girl: The pelvic pain report*, p. 18.

30 Steege and Siedhoff, 'Chronic pelvic pain'.

31 Alison Hey-Cunningham, from her presentation to the EndoActive conference, Sydney, 2015.

32 IASP, 'Endometriosis and its association with other painful conditions', Fact Sheet, Global Year Against Pain in Women, International Association for the Study of Pain, 2007, <www.iasp-pain.org/Advocacy/Content.aspx?ItemNumber=1107>.

33 'Falling', *Sharp Objects*, HBO, 2018. Produced by David Auge, directed by Jean-Marc Vallée. Based on the book *Sharp Objects* by Gillian Flynn.

34 Paul Ingraham, 'Sensitization in Chronic Pain', *Pain Science*, 29 March 2019, <www.painscience.com/articles/central-sensitization.php>.

35 Coxon, Horne and Vincent, 'Pathophysiology of endometriosis-associated pain'.

36 Coxon, Horne and Vincent, 'Pathophysiology of endometriosis-associated pain'.

37 Evans, Brooks, Esterman et al., 'The comorbidities of dysmenorrhea'.

38 Evans, Brooks, Esterman et al., 'The comorbidities of dysmenorrhea'.

39 Steege and Siedhoff, 'Chronic pelvic pain'.

40 K.N. Khan, A. Fujishita, K. Hiraki et al., 'Bacterial contamination hypothesis: A new concept in endometriosis', *Reproductive Medicine and Biology*, 2018, 17(2): 125–33, doi: 10.1002/rmb2.12083.

41 K. Vincent, C. Warnaby, C.J. Stagg et al., 'Dysmenorrhoea is associated with central changes in otherwise healthy women', *Pain*, 2011, 152(9): 1966–75, doi: 10.1016/j.pain.2011.03.029.

42 Vincent, Warnaby, Stagg et al., 'Dysmenorrhoea is associated with central changes in otherwise healthy women'.

43 Gemma Hardi, Susan Evans and Meredith Craigie, 'A possible link between dysmenorrhoea and the development of chronic pelvic pain', *Australian and New Zealand Journal of Obstetrics and Gynaecology*, 2014, 54: 593–6, doi: 10.1111/ajo.12274.

44 Hoffman and Tarzian, 'The Girl Who Cried Pain', p. 23.

45 Pelvic Pain Steering Committee, *The $6 Billion Woman and the $600 Million Girl: The pelvic pain report*, p. 26.

46 M. Parker, A. Sneddon and P. Arbon, 'The menstrual disorder of teenagers (MDOT) study: Determining typical menstrual patterns and menstrual disturbance in a large population-based study of Australian teenagers', *BJOG: An International Journal of Obstetrics & Gynaecology*, 2010, 117: 185–92, doi: 10.1111/j.1471-0528.2009.02407.x.

47 John Guillebaud, cited in Olivia Goldhill, 'Period pain can be "almost as bad as a heart attack"', *Quartz*, 16 February 2016, <https://qz.com/611774/period-pain-can-be-as-bad-as-a-heart-attack-so-why-arent-we-researching-how-to-treat-it/>.

48 A.M. Aloisi, V. Bachiocco, A. Constantino et al., 'Cross-sex hormone administration changes pain in transsexual women and men', *Pain*, 2007, 132 (Suppl. 1): S60–S67, doi: 10.1016/j.pain.2007.02.006.

49 H.D. White, L.A.J. Brown, R.J. Gyurik et al., 'Treatment of pain in fibromyalgia patients with testosterone gel: Pharmacokinetics and clinical response', *International Immunopharmacology*, 2015, 27(2): 249–56, doi: 10.1016/j.intimp.2015.05.016.

50 IASP, 'Sex differences in pain: Basic science findings', Fact Sheet, Global Year Against Pain in Women, International Association for the Study of Pain, 2007, <www.iasp-pain.org/Advocacy/Content.aspx?ItemNumber=1107>

51 Pelvic Pain Steering Committee, *The $6 Billion Woman and the $600 Million Girl: The pelvic pain report*, p. 12.

Chapter 7

1   WHO, 'Maternal and reproductive health: Global health observatory data', World Health Organization, <www.who.int/gho/maternal_health/en/>.

2   Linda Villarosa, 'Why America's black mothers and babies are in a life-or-death crisis', *New York Times Magazine*, 11 April 2018, <www.nytimes.com/2018/04/11/magazine/black-mothers-babies-death-maternal-mortality.html>.

3   Villarosa, 'Why America's black mothers and babies are in a life or death crisis'.

4   AIHW, 'Maternal deaths in Australia 2012–2014', Australian Institute of Health and Welfare, 8 December 2017, <www.aihw.gov.au/reports/mothers-babies/maternal-deaths-in-australia-2012-2014/contents/risk-factors-for-maternal-death>.

5   S. Kildea, S. Hickey, C. Nelson et al., 'Birthing on Country (in our community): A case study of engaging stakeholders and developing a best practice Indigenous maternity service in an urban setting', *Australian Health Review*, 2018, 42(2): 230–88, doi: 10.1071/AH16218.

6   Atul Gawande, 'The score: How childbirth went industrial', *New Yorker*, 1 October 2006, <www.newyorker.com/magazine/2006/10/09/the-score>.

7   Wenger, 'You've come a long way, baby'.

8   G.E. Ratcliffe, M.W. Enns, S.L. Belik and J. Sareen, 'Chronic pain conditions and suicidal ideation and suicide attempts: An epidemiologic perspective', *The Clinical Journal of Pain*, 2008, 24(3): 204–10, doi: 10.1097/AJP.0b013e31815ca2a3.

9   Lena Dunham, Instagram, 7 October 2018, <www.instagram.com/p/BomwRFNlqsh/?utm_source=ig_embed&utm_campaign=embed_loading_state_control>.

10 *Gaga: Five Foot Two*. Directed by Chris Moukarbel, Live Nations Productions, Mermaid Films, Permanent Wave, 2017.

11 Jonathan Van Meter, 'Lady Gaga opens up about *A Star Is Born*, MeToo, and a decade in pop', *Vogue*, 10 September 2018, <www.vogue.com/article/lady-gaga-vogue-cover-october-2018-issue>.

12 Selena Gomez, Instagram, 14 September 2017, <www.instagram.com/p/BZBHr4Pg5Wd/?utm_source=ig_embed>.

13 Evelyn Wang, 'Selena Gomez said her lupus was "life-or-death" before her kidney transplant', *TeenVogue*, 21 November 2017, <www.teenvogue.com/story/selena-gomez-speech-lupus-research-alliance-breaking-through-gala>.

14 Melody Chiu, 'Selena Gomez taking time off after dealing with "anxiety, pain attacks and depression" due to her lupus diagnosis', *People*, 30 August 2016.

15 Karen Crouse, 'Williams says she struggled with fatigue for years', *New York Times*, 1 September 2011, <www.nytimes.com/2011/09/02/sports/tennis/2011-us-open-venus-williams-describes-fights-with-fatigue.html>.

16 Manne, *Down Girl*, pp. 249–56.

17 Manne, *Down Girl*, p. 266.

18 Manne, *Down Girl*, p. 236.

19 S. Simoens, G. Dunselman, C. Dirksen et al., 'The burden of endometriosis: Costs and quality of life of women with endometriosis and treated in referral

centres', *Human Reproduction*, 2012, 27(5): 1292–9, doi: 10.1093/humrep/des073.

20 T. D'Hooge, C.D. Dirksen, G.A.J, Dunselman et al., 'The costs of endometriosis: It's the economy, stupid', *Fertility & Sterility*, 2012, 98(3): S218–S219, doi: 10.1016/j.fertnstert.2012.07.791.

21 CPRA White Paper, *Impact of Chronic Overlapping Pain Conditions*, p. 21.

22 IASP, 'Endometriosis and its association with other painful conditions'.

23 N. Sinai, S.D. Cleary, M.L. Ballweg et al., 'High rates of autoimmune and endocrine disorders, fibromyalgia, chronic fatigue syndrome and atopic diseases among women with endometriosis: survey analysis', *Human Reproduction*, 2002, 17(10): 2715–24, <www.ncbi.nlm.nih.gov/pubmed/12351553>.

24 CPRA White Paper, *Impact of Chronic Overlapping Pain Conditions*, p. 11.

25 IASP, 'Vulvodynia', Fact Sheet, Global Year Against Pain in Women, International Association for the Study of Pain, 2007, <www.iasp-pain.org/Advocacy/Content.aspx?ItemNumber=1107>.

26 'Vulval pain', Pelvic Pain Support Network, <www.pelvicpain.org.uk/conditions/vulval-pain/>.

27 IASP, 'Fibromyalgia syndrome (FMS)', Fact Sheet, Global Year Against Pain in Women, International Association for the Study of Pain, 2007, <www.iasp-pain.org/Advocacy/Content.aspx?ItemNumber=1107>.

28 IASP, 'Fibromyalgia syndrome (FMS)'.

29 IASP, 'Fibromyalgia syndrome (FMS)'.

30 CPRA White Paper, *Impact of Chronic Overlapping Pain Conditions*, p. 21.

31 IASP, 'Fibromyalgia syndrome (FMS)'.

32 CDC, 'Myalgic encephalomyelitis/Chronic fatigue syndrome: Information for health providers', Centers for Disease Control and Prevention, <www.cdc.gov/me-cfs/healthcare-providers/index.html>.

33 CPRA White Paper, *Impact of Chronic Overlapping Pain Conditions*, p. 11.

34 'Beyond Myalgic encephalomyelitis/Chronic fatigue syndrome: Redefining an illness', Institute of Medicine of the National Academies, 10 February 2015, <www.nationalacademies.org/hmd/Reports/2015/ME-CFS.aspx>.

35 CPRA White Paper, *Impact of Chronic Overlapping Pain Conditions*, p. 13.

36 Shuu-Jiun Wang, Ping-Kun Chen and Jong-Ling Fuh, 'Comorbidities of migraine', *Frontiers in Neurology*, 2010, 1: 16, doi: 10.3389/fneur.2010.00016.

37 R.A. Deyo, Samuel F. Dworkin, Dagmar Amtmann et al., *Report of the Task Force on Research Standards for Chronic Low-Back Pain*, 2013, <http://painconsortium.nih.gov/NIH_Pain_Programs/Task_Force/cLBP_RTF_FullReport.pdf>.

38 CPRA White Paper, *Impact of Chronic Overlapping Pain Conditions*, p. 12.

39 Jonathan Lomas, Taylan Gurgenci, Christopher Jackson and Duncan Campbell, 'Temporomandibular dysfunction', *Australia Journal of General Practice*, 2018, 47(4), <www1.racgp.org.au/ajgp/2018/april/temporomandibular-dysfunction>.

40 S. Sharma, D.S. Gupta, U.S. Pal and S.K. Jurel, 'Etiological factors of

temporomandibular joint disorders', *National Journal of Maxillofacial Surgery*, 2011, 2(2): 116–19, doi: 10.4103/0975-5950.94463.

41 CPRA White Paper, *Impact of Chronic Overlapping Pain Conditions*, p. 11.

42 H. Dahan, Y. Shir, A. Velly and P. Allison, 'Specific and number of comorbidities are associated with increased levels of temporomandibular pain intensity and duration', *Journal of Headache and Pain*, 2015, 16: 528, doi: 10.1186/s10194-015-0528-2.

43 DeLisa Fairweather and Noel R. Rose, 'Women and autoimmune diseases', *Emerging Infectious Diseases*, 2004, 10(11): 2005–11, doi: 10.3201/eid1011.040367.

44 Sandberg, cited in Saini, *Inferior*, p. 49.

45 P. Panopalis, J. Yazdany, J.Z. Gillis et al., 'Health care costs and costs associated with changes in work productivity among persons with systemic lupus erythematosus', *Arthritis and Rheumatism*, 2008, 59(12): 1788–95, doi: 10.1002/art.24063.

46 LFA, 'Lupus facts and statistics', National Resource Center on Lupus, Lupus Foundation of America, <www.lupus.org/resources/lupus-facts-and-statistics>.

47 ACR, 'Rheumatoid arthritis', American College of Rheumatology, <www.rheumatology.org/I-Am-A/Patient-Caregiver/Diseases-Conditions/Rheumatoid-Arthritis>.

48 AIHW, 'Rheumatoid arthritis', Australia Institute of Health and Welfare, <www.aihw.gov.au/reports/chronic-musculoskeletal-conditions/rheumatoid-arthritis/contents/who-gets-rheumatoid-arthritis>.

49 NRAS, 'What is RA?', National Rheumatoid Arthritis Society, <www.nras.org.uk/what-is-ra-article>.

50 Steven E. Carsons and Bhupendra C. Patel, 'Sjögren syndrome', StatPearls Publishing: Treasure Island, FL, 2019, <www.ncbi.nlm.nih.gov/books/NBK431049/>.

51 'Sjögren's syndrome', Garvan Institute of Medical Research, <www.garvan.org.au/research/diseases/sjogrens-syndrome>.

Chapter 8

1 King, in *Hysteria Beyond Freud*, p. 17.

2 Roni Caryn Rabin, 'Health researchers will get $10.1 million to counter gender bias in studies', *New York Times*, 23 September 2014, <www.nytimes.com/2014/09/23/health/23gender.html>.

3 Young, Fisher and Kirkman, 'Do mad people get endo or does endo make you mad?', p. 5.

4 'Women's health: Report of the Public Health Service Task Force on Women's Health Issues', *Public Health Reports*, 1985, 100(1): 73–106.

5 Dusenbery, *Doing Harm*, p. 25.

6 Dusenbery, *Doing Harm*, p. 25.

7 S.K. Lee, 'Sex as an important biological variable in biomedical research', *BMB Reports*, 2018, 51(4), 167–73, doi: 10.5483/BMBRep.2018.51.4.034.

8   Leslie Laurence and Beth Weinhouse, *Outrageous Practices: How gender bias threatens women's health,* Rutgers University Press: New Brunswick, NJ, 1997 [1994], p. 71.

9   A.K. Beery and I. Zucker, 'Sex bias in neuroscience and biomedical research', *Neuroscience and biobehavioral reviews,* 2010, 35(3): 565–72, doi: 10.1016/j.neubiorev.2010.07.002.

10 Isaac Baker Brown, *On the Curability of Certain Forms of Insanity, Epilepsy, Catalepsy, and Hysteria in Females,* Robert Hardwicke: London, 1866.

11 McRae, *Unwell,* pp. 275–6.

12 McRae, *Unwell,* p. 276.

13 McRae, *Unwell,* p. 276.

14 CWLU Her Story Project, 'Sterilization abuse: A task for the women's movement', <http://freedomarchives.org/Documents/Finder/DOC46_scans/46.SterilizationAbuseWomenTheFacts.pdf>.

15 Phoebe Friesen, 'Educational pelvic exams on anesthetized women: Why consent matters', *Bioethics,* 2018, 32(5): 298–307, doi: 10.1111/bioe.12441.

16 Yvette Coldicott, Britt-Ingjerd Nesheim, Jane MacDougall et al., 'The ethics of intimate examinations: Teaching tomorrow's doctors', *BMJ,* 2003, 326: 97, doi: 10.1136/bmj.326.7380.97.

17 Coldicott, Nesheim, MacDougall et al., 'The ethics of intimate examinations'.

18 C.E. Rees and L.V. Monrouxe, 'Medical students learning intimate examinations without valid consent: A multicentre study', *Medical Education,* 2011, 45(3): 261–72, doi: 10.1111/j.1365-2923.2010.03911.x.

19 CPRA White Paper, *Impact of Chronic Overlapping Pain Conditions,* p. 15.

20 'National Pain Strategy: Pain management for all Australians', Pain Australia, 2011, <www.painaustralia.org.au/static/uploads/files/national-pain-strategy-2011-wfvjawttsanq.pdf>.

21 CPPC, 'A report of the Pain Summit 2011', Chronic Pain Policy Coalition, pp. 8–9, <www.britishpainsociety.org/static/uploads/resources/files/members_articles_pain_summit_report.pdf>.

22 Greenspan, Craft, LeResche et al., 'Studying sex and gender differences in pain and analgesia'.

23 Greenspan, Craft, LeResche et al., 'Studying sex and gender differences in pain and analgesia'.

24 Pelvic Pain Steering Committee, *The $6 Billion Woman and the $600 Million Girl: The pelvic pain report,* p. 19.

25 Pelvic Pain Steering Committee, *The $6 Billion Woman and the $600 Million Girl: The pelvic pain report,* p. 8.

26 Pelvic Pain Steering Committee, *The $6 Billion Woman and the $600 Million Girl: The pelvic pain report,* p. 8.

27 AIHW, *Australia's Young People 2003: Their health and wellbeing,* Australian Institute of Health and Welfare, 2003, 1–422, <www.aihw.gov.au/publication-detail/?id=6442467534>.

28 Pelvic Pain Steering Committee, *The $6 Billion Woman and the $600 Million Girl: The pelvic pain report*, p. 25.

29 National Health and Medicine Research Council figures, email to the author, 2 January 2019.

30 CPRA White Paper, *Impact of Chronic Overlapping Pain Conditions*, p. 19.

31 CPRA White Paper, *Impact of Chronic Overlapping Pain Conditions*, p. 10.

32 Often a complication of shingles, postherpetic neuralgia affects skin and nerve fibres, creating a burning sensation that lasts after the shingles rash and blisters have cleared up. Capsaicin is the active ingredient in chilli peppers that makes your mouth feel hot. There is growing evidence that it can ease neuropathic pain when formulated into a cream or patch that can be applied to skin. It's also been used to treat patients with fibromyalgia, rheumatoid arthritis and osteoarthritis, migraines, headaches and muscle strain.

33 Institute of Medicine (US) Committee on Advancing Pain Research, Care, and Education, *Relieving Pain in America*, p. 224.

34 Institute of Medicine (US) Committee on Advancing Pain Research, Care, and Education, *Relieving Pain in America*, p. 225.

35 NHMRC, email response of 2 January 2019 to my question.

36 Institute of Medicine (US) Committee on Advancing Pain Research, Care, and Education, *Relieving Pain in America*, p. 252.

37 Apoorva Mandavilli, 'H.I.V. is reported cured in a second patient, a milestone in the global AIDS epidemic', *New York Times*, 4 March 2019, <www.nytimes.com/2019/03/04/health/aids-cure-london-patient.html>.

38 June Gibbs Brown, 'Audit of Costs Charged to the Chronic Fatigue Syndrome Program at the Centers for Disease Control and Prevention,' Department of Health and Human Services, 10 May 1999 <https://oig.hhs.gov/oas/reports/region4/49804226.pdf>

39 Dusenbery, *Doing Harm*, p. 266.

40 Dusenbery, *Doing Harm*, p. 264.

41 P. Vercellini, L. Buggio, E. Somigliana et al., 'Attractiveness of women with rectovaginal endometriosis: A case-control study', *Fertility and Sterility*, 2013, 99(1): 212–18, doi: 10.1016/j.fertnstert.2012.08.039.

42 Jacqueline Howard, '10 top questions you had for Dr Google in 2018', CNN, 27 December 2018, <https://edition.cnn.com/2018/12/21/health/health-questions-2018-google-explainer/index.html>.

43 Greg Hunt, '$10 million funding boost for endometriosis research and awareness', Minister for Health, 9 April 2019, <www.health.gov.au/internet/ministers/publishing.nsf/Content/health-mediarel-yr2019-hunt124.htm>.

44 Orrin Hatch, 'Orrin Hatch: This is nothing short of a public health emergency', CNN, 28 March 2018, <https://edition.cnn.com/2018/03/27/opinions/endometriosis-start-a-conversation-hatch-opinion/index.html>.

Epilogue

1 John A. Astin, 'Why patients use alternative medicine: Results of a national survey', *Journal of the American Medical Association*, 1998, 279(19): 1548–53.

INDEX

Page numbers in *italics* refer to figures

Abbott, Chloe 184
Abbott, Jason 192
abortion 165
acute pain 222–3, 232, 255
adenomyosis 3–4, 6, 152, 217–20
African-American women 81–2, 121–2, 139, 257–8, 261, 298–301
age and ageing 62, 65, 68, 77–8, 296
All-Party Parliamentary Group on Women's Health (UK) 191, 194, 199, 315
alternative therapies 320–1
American College of Rheumatology 275
amitriptyline 196, 248, 262
anaesthesia 100
anal sex 141–2, 144, 156
Anderson, Gillian 63
Ansari, Aziz 126, 135
anxiety 115, 227, 262, 320
Aristotle 64, 292
arousal 31, 130–1
arousal non-concordance 131
arthritis 309
Asian women 122–3
Australasian Menopause Society 75
autoimmune conditions 8–9, 163, 261–2, 265, 283–91
Ayers, Beverley 62

bacteria 249–50
Badham, Van 83–4
Baker Brown, Isaac 100–1, 298
Ballweg, Mary Lou 17
Bancroft, John 131
Bateman, Lucinda 314
Battey, Robert 101, 298–9
Beard, George 103, 116
Beery, Annaliese 297
Bendelow, Gillian 234
Benjamin, Marina 64, 78

bikini approach, to women's health 14, 261
bioidentical hormone therapy 75–6
birth control movement 301
birth control pills *see* contraceptive pills
black women *see* African-American women; Indigenous women
Booysen, Nina 128, 132–3, 142, 144–6, 156
borderline personality disorder 113, 115, 159–62, 173–4, 176
Boshoff, Alison 122
the brain 9, 49, 67, 129, 131–2, 229, 231, 244
Breuer, Josef 109–11
British Menopause Society 75
British Society for Gynaecological Endoscopy 315
Brown, Isaac *see* Baker Brown, Isaac
Burrows, George Man 99

cardiovascular disease *see* heart disease
Carter, Robert Brudenell 97–8
'catastrophising' 226–7
celebrities, as advocates 63, 263–5, 316–17
Centers for Disease Control and Prevention (US) 276, 313
central sensitisation 240
cervix 22, 26–8, 52
Charcot, Jean-Martin 105–9, *108*
Cheyne, George 93, 103, 116
Chiaramonte, Gabrielle 176
children, pain in 225, *225*, 228, 306
Chinese medicine 72
chronic diseases 190, 195–6
chronic fatigue syndrome 9–10, 174, 195, 238–9, *270*, 276–7, 313–14, 320
chronic low back pain 10, 239, *270*, 279–80

chronic overlapping pain conditions 10, 239, 261, 270, *270*, 307–8
chronic pain
  alternative therapies 320–1
  chronic pain conditions *270*, 270–83
  funding for 9–10, 303, 310–13
  lack of training to deal with 176
  male bias in research 14–15
  rates of by age and gender 225, *225*
  relation to mental health 261–2
  treatment of 248
  understanding chronic pain 222–4
  in women 164, 224–35
  see also chronic pelvic pain;
    endometriosis; period pain
Chronic Pain Research Alliance (US) 10, 239, 261, 272, 280, 306–8
chronic pelvic pain 235–55
  association with hysteria 162
  as a condition in its own right 270, *270*
  funding for 310
  lack of acknowledgement of by government 305–6
  and Medicare 189–90
  pain relief 54, 170
  painful intercourse as a result of 144, 146
  surgery for 193–4
  treatment of 196
  in women 225
chronic tension-type headache 10, 239, *270*, 278–9
cisgender women 17–18
Clark, Edward 104
Clayton, Janine Austin 14, 293
clinical trials 14, 296–8
clitoral hood 32, *33*
clitoridectomy 100–1
clitoris 36–9, *37*, 100, 138
coercion *see* sexual domination
Cohn, Shannon 17, 317
Come as You Are . . . (Nagoski) 124–5, 130, 133–4
Complaints and Disorders (Ehrenreich and English) 96, 146–7
confirmation bias 56
consent 126, 130–1, 142, 301–2
contraceptive pills 54, 120, 164–5, 254
corpus luteum 50–1
Coxon, Lydia 228, 247

Craigie, Meredith 251
Crohn's disease 285
cutaneous lupus erythematosus 285

Darwin, Charles 103, 135
de Beauvoir, Simone 76
deep-infiltrating endometriosis 195, 217
Dent, Georgina 181
depression 8, 67–8, 77, 113, 115, 174, 227, 262
Descartes, René 231–2
desire 130–3
diagnosis 201–2, 251, 263
dialectical behaviour therapy 159
diclofenac 54
'difficult' women 4, 47, 80, 85, 88, 162, 167–8, 171, 173
disadvantaged women 206–12
'doctor-shopping' 232
doctors *see* medical profession
Dodsworth, Laura 34
Down Girl: The logic of misogyny (Manne) 119, 123, 151, 172, 265
Dunham, Lena 121, 192, 263, 267–8, 316
Dusenbery, Maya 164, 198, 202, 232, 296, 313–14
dysmenorrhea 248, 250
dyspareunia 127

Edes, R.T. 102
education 11, 46, 104, 143, 175–8, 181–2, 252
eggs (oocytes) 23–4, 49–50, 52, 65
Ehlers-Danlos syndrome 263, 269
Ehrenreich, Barbara 96, 99, 146–7
emotional intelligence 77
emotions, and PMS 56–8
Endep 248
EndoActive 3, 169
endocrine system 294
endometriosis
  advocacy for 10
  association with hysteria 13, 162, 167–8, 175
  as a chronic condition 270, *270*
  cost of 254, 271–2
  defined 6
  and fertility 152–3, 169–70
  funding for 4, 314–16
  obstacles to therapy 5

overview of 271–3
pain of 1–3, 9, 148, 170–1, 192–3, 199,
   217–18, 220–2, 238–9, 246–7, 263
in the *Pelvic Pain Report* 305
prevalence of 4, 271
retrograde menstruation theory 246
surgery for 191–4, 217–19, 262
treatment in the public system 189–91
treatment of 196, 272
UK guide on management of 315
Endometriosis Association (US) 17
endometrium 6, 26, 50–3
energy conservation theory 103–4
English, Deirdre 96, 99, 146–7
Erikson, Erik 112
Evans, Susan 53, 148, 151, 166, 173, 176,
   191–2, 198–9, 240–9, 291, 310–11,
   314
Eve Appeal 11, 21, 29, 47
evolutionary biology 61, 135–6
Expert Patient Program 190

Fairweather, Claire 143–4, 160–1,
   168–9, 171, 176, 189–90, 192
fallopian tubes *22*, 25
family violence 158–9
female genital mutilation 137–8
female reproductive system *21*, 21–41,
   22, 98, 104, 243–4, *244*, 256
female sexuality 117–57
femininity 56, 119, 152
feminism 112–14
fertilisation, of eggs 50–3
fertility 52, 152–4, 168–9
fibroids 191
fibromyalgia 9–10, 174–5, 195, 225, 228,
   238–9, 242, 263–4, *270*, 274–6, 309
FIFE patients 201
fistula 298–9
Fleabag (television program) 63, 121, 236
follicle-stimulating hormone 49–50
follicles 23–4, 48–9, 65
follicular phase *48*, 48–9
Food and Drug Administration (US)
   70–1, 74, 296–7
food intolerances 243
foot binding 137
frailty, as a beauty ideal *147*, 147–8
Franklin, Benjamin 94–5
free association 111
Freedman, Sylvia 169–70

Freud, Sigmund 12, 95, 105, 109–12
Friedan, Betty 78
Friesen, Phoebe 301
fruit flies 135–6
funding, for research 272, 274–5, 277,
   279–83, 286, 289, 307, 309–17

Gawande, Atul 260
gender 9, 17–18, 229–34, 242, 253, 261,
   304–5
general practice 184–5, 188
genital mutilation 137–8
genitalia, describing 31–2
George, Rose 77
'The girl who cried pain' 233–5, 252
glans clitoris *33*, 36–8
gonads 23
Grace, Victoria 234
'grandmother theory' of menopause 61,
   76
Graves' disease 289–91
Groopman, Jerome 201–2, 205–6
Guillebaud, John 253
Gulf War syndrome 113
gynaecology 95, 98–102, 191–5, 201,
   298–302

Haden, Sir Francis Seymour 100
Hailes, Jean 316
Hamer, Fannie Lou 300
Hamilton, A.M. 102
Hardi, Gemma 251
Hashimoto's thyroiditis 289–91
Hawkes, Kristen 61
headache *see* chronic tension-type
   headache; migraine
heart disease 6–7, 14, 176–7, 200, 296
'heartsink patients' 174, 176, 188
Hefner, Hugh 120–1
Herbenick, Debby 127
Hey-Cunningham, Alison 238
Hippocrates 86
Hirsch, Afua 121–2
Hoffman, Diane 233, 252
homosexuality 138
honour killings 137, 140
hormone replacement therapy 60, 68,
   71–6, 309
hormones 12, 24, 53, 56–8, 253, 294
Horne, Andrew 247
hot flushes 67

Howell, Mary C. 197
Hunt, Greg 315–16
Hutchinson, Mark 15, 229–32, 241, 245–6
hymen 39–41, *40*
hyperthyroidism 290–1
hypnosis 107, 109, 111
hypochondria 8, 13, 106, 172, 205, 239
hypothyroidism 290–1
hysterectomy 4, 6, 65, 192, 300–1
hysteria 12–13, 80–116, 160–2, 166–75,
    177, 203–4, 226–8, 263

ibuprofen 54
illness, as control 146–57
immune system *see* autoimmune
    conditions
Indigenous Australians 286
Indigenous women 139–40, 172,
    206–12, 258–61
industrialisation 116
infant mortality 207, 257–9
Inferior (Saini) 61, 135–6, 242, 284
inflammation 245–7
Institute of Medicine (US) 224, 310
International Association for the Study of
    Pain 222, 225, 232–5, 273–4
International Menopause Society 75
interstitial cystitis 9–10, 238–9, 243,
    270, *270*, 281–2
intrauterine devices 54, 186–8, *187*, 301
irritable bowel syndrome 9, 206, 225,
    238–9, 242–3, 251, 270, *270*, 280–1
IVF 152–3

Janssen, Eric 131
Johnson & Johnson 154–6
Johnston, Casey 186
Johnston, Grace 77
Jones, Rebecca Manson 212
Jones, Trina 81
Jorden, Edward 88–9

Kelly, Howard 102
King, Helen 86
Kundera, Milan 12, 20

labia *22*, 29–30, 32–5
labia majora 32, *33*, 34–5
labia minora 32, *33*, 34–5
labiaplasty 33, 142
Lady Gaga 263–4

Lamnisos, Athena 21, 29–30
laparoscopic surgery 192, 194, 217,
    219–20
Laurence, Leslie 297
Leonard, Rosemary 67
lesbians 71, 139
LGBTI+ people 261, 313
libido, lack of 69–70
life expectancy 10, 163–4, 207
listening, to patients 196–206, 319, 321
London 91
Loofbourow, Lili 126–7
love sickness 89
low back pain *see* chronic low back pain
'low mood' 67–8
lubrication 31, 71
lunatic asylums 95
lupus 264–5, 285–7, 289, 291
Lupus Research Alliance 264–5
luteal phase *48*, 49–51
luteinising hormones 49, 50

McCartney, Jamie 34
McKay, Sarah 55
McMullin, Gabrielle 178–9
McRae, Mike 80–2, 138, 300
The Madness of Women (Ussher) 113–14,
    124, 159–60
Madonna–whore complex 124, 135
male bias, in research 14–15, 230,
    292–8, 304–5
Managing the Monstrous Feminine (Ussher)
    57, 77–8
Manne, Kate 119, 123, 151, 172, 265–8
Marston, Cecily 141
Martin, Emily 49–50
masculinity 134
masturbation 100, 117, 128–9, 143
maternal mortality 207, 257–9
Matthews, K.A. 62
Maudsley, Henry 104
medical menopause 65
medical profession
    anger towards 319
    Cartesian model of medicine 231
    construction of female sexuality 118
    control of women's reproductive rights
        118, 164–5
    culture of 178–83
    diagnosis of borderline personality
        disorder 159–62

dismissal of women's symptoms by
4, 6, 8–11, 22, 114, 171, 196–8,
203–12, 226–8, 232, 235
disparities in treatment of women
15–17, 44, 176–7, 233–4, 252,
294–5
education to treat period pain seriously
252
on endometriosis 4, 13
female doctors 183–5
feudal wars within 180
as guardians of women's interests 100,
102
historical development of 96
hysteria narratives by 12–13, 162,
166–75, 226–7, 263
importance of listening to patients
196–206, 319, 321
income disparity by gender 183, 185
male bias in 11, 99, 176, 200, 292–8,
304–5
medical education 175–8, 181–2
medical errors 205
on menopause 59–61
mental health of doctors 181–2
need for change in 318–21
pelvic examinations without consent
301–2
perception of menstruation 45
perception of women and their bodies
292–5
power imbalance in doctor/patient
relationship 172
racial bias within 206–11, 257–8
reaction to vaginal mesh scandal
156–7
reluctance of women to report
symptoms to 21–2, 47, 235
sexism in health care 162–3, 165–6
talking about sex 145–6, 157
undervaluing of women's skills 183–9
Medical Research Future Fund 316
'medically unexplained symptoms' 13,
114, 198, 232
Medicare 185–6, 188–91, 193–4
Meldrum, Marcia L. 232
men
control over women 118, 151–2
experience of pain 234, 253–4
fertility of 153–4
heart disease 6–7

hormonal changes in later life 65, 71
hysteria in 90, 93, 102–3, 108
immune responses 8
male bias in research 14–15, 230,
292–8, 304–5
male protectiveness 148–51, 266
in the medical profession 99, 180
prevalence of chronic pain 225, 225–6
sexuality of 120–7, 133–6, 138–41
menopause 58–79
attitudes to 76–9
biology of 64–6
differing experiences of 77–8
as a disease 60, 72–3, 78
grandmother theory of 61, 76
impacts of 66–71
invisibility after 16
myths about 12, 59–62
in other cultures 62
see also hormone replacement therapy
menopause cafes 64
Menstrual Education 252
menstruation 42–58
expense of 43–4
menstrual cycle 23–4, 26, 30, 47–51,
48, 56
myths surrounding 42–3, 45–6
retrograde menstruation 246
taboos surrounding 12, 42–3, 45–7,
118
see also period pain
mental health, of doctors 181–2
mental illness 16, 102, 113
Mesmer, Franz Anton 94–5
#MeToo movement 120, 126, 135, 145,
202
Micale, Mark 108
microglia 15, 230
midwives 99
migraine 9–10, 225, 238–9, 270, 278–9,
308
Million Women Study (UK) 73, 75
misogyny 119, 172, 265, 267–8
Mitchell, Silas Weir 104–5
Mohamed, Janine 258–9
monogamy 136–7
mons pubis 32, 33
Mood in Daily Life study 57
mood swings 56–7, 67–8
Moore, Suzanne 63
morning-after pill 165

mound of Venus 32
Munthe, Axel 107
myalgic encephalomyelitis 9–10, 276

Nagoski, Emily 123–6, 129–35
naproxen 54
National Academy for Medicine (US) 223
National Health and Medical Research
    Council (Australia) 272, 274–5,
    277, 279–83, 286, 289, 307, 310
National Health Service (UK) 190, 195,
    198, 315
National Institute for Health and Care
    Excellence (UK) 277, 315
National Institute of Medicine (US) 277
National Institutes of Health (US) 14,
    230, 239, 272, 274–5, 277, 279–83,
    288, 297, 303, 311
National Pain Strategy (2010) 303, 306
National Pain Summit (Australia) 303
National Pain Summit (UK) 303–4
neurasthenia 103–5
neurology 95, 101–9
night sweats 67
nonsteroidal anti-inflammatory drugs
    53–4
North American Menopause Society 75

obstetrics 99, 260
O'Connell, Helen 38
oestradiol 24
oestrogen 24, 30, 48–9, 55, 65–74
Office of Research on Women's Health
    (US) 14, 56, 261
OMGYes 128–9
oophorectomy 65, 101–2, 106
opioids 54, 175, 211
Orady, Mona 201
oral sex 41, 144
Orange is the New Black (television
    program) 36
orgasms 37, 125, 128
Osler, Sir William 202
osteoarthritis 225
ovaries 22, 23–4, 101
ovulation 49, 65
ovulation pain 19–20
ownership 148–9

pain 213–55
    assessment of 312

central sensitisation 240
    in children 225, 225, 228
    defined 222
    disparities in treatment of women
        233–4, 252
    gender differences 9, 18, 229–34, 242,
        304
    invisible pain 242–3
    language to describe 173
    pain sensitisation 250
    pelvic pain 235–55
    relation to mood 172
    research on 15
    sexual pain 126–7, 143–4, 154–7
    types of 222–3
    underinvestment in research 303–17,
        312
    understanding pain 222–4
    in women 10–11
    women's coping strategies 234
    see also acute pain; chronic pain
pain relief 53–4, 196, 222–3, 248, 262
painful bladder syndrome 9–10, 238–9,
    243, 270, 270, 281–2
pap smears 185–6, 189
parenthood, delaying of 153–4
Park, Patricia 122
Parker, Melissa 252
patriarchy 56, 95, 114, 125, 134, 138,
    146
pelvic floor 244
pelvic pain see chronic pelvic pain;
    period pain
Pelvic Pain Foundation of Australia
    53–4, 241, 252
Perel, Esther 138, 140–1, 145
period pain 47, 53–4, 199, 214, 217–18,
    250–3
periods see menstruation
pharmaceutical companies 309
physiotherapy 195–6, 218, 262
Pinker, Steven 136
Plan International Australia 45–6
Plato 87
pleasure givers, women as 123–4
pleasure, sexual 129–31
pop culture, sex in 121
pornography 121, 124, 140, 142
post-traumatic stress disorder 113, 115,
    158
poverty 43–4, 91, 261, 300–1

power relations 119, 138
pre-mentrual syndrome 55–8
pregnancy 4, 51–3, 76, 170
Price, Steve 83–4
progesterone 24, 49–51, 55, 65
progestin 54, 73
prostaglandins 53–4
psychiatry 95, 113
psychoanalysis 109–10, 112
psychological trauma 158–9

racial stereotyping 81, 211
racism 121, 139, 211–12, 257–8, 261
Radcliffe, John 92
'raging hormones' 58, 72, 85
Ramey, Estelle 70, 72
Rankin, Tom 45
Ray, Keisha 211
Raz, Shlomo 156
reflex theory 99
Reilly, Caroline 236
Relieving Pain in America (report) 10, 224, 261, 263, 303, 309, 311
religion 118–19, 140
repressed memories 110–11
reproductive system *see* female reproductive system
research 13–15, 164, 230, 293–317
responsive desire 133–4
rest cure 104–5
retrograde menstruation 246
Reuben, David 59–60
rheumatoid arthritis 9, 225, 242, 287–9, 291
Romans, Sarah 56–7
Rooney, Sally 116
Rosenberg, Charles 98
Roter, Debra 201–2
Rousseau, George 85, 87, 90–1, 106, 113, 115
Royal Australasian College of Surgeons 179

Saini, Angela 61, 135–6, 242, 284
Saldanha, Anita 142–3, 159, 172, 174, 176, 179, 188–9
Sandberg, Kathryn 284
sanitary products 43–4
Scelza, Brooke 136
Scotland 43
Scull, Andrew 86, 109–11, 113

sex and sexuality 123–36
    after menopause 69–71
    education about 143, 145
    illness as control 146–57
    patriarchal standards of 125
    pleasure, desire and arousal 129–34
    in pop culture 121
    reduced incidence of sex 141
    relation to power 119, 138
    repression of female sexuality 117–20
    research on 128–9
    sex as a method of control 136–44
    sex distinguished from gender 17–18, 85
    sexual dysfunction 146
    sexual health 144–6
    sexual pain 126–7, 143–4, 154–7
    stereotypes of 117–18, 121–2, 124
sex chromosomes 254
sex hormones 24, 62
sexism 15, 118–19, 162–3, 165–6, 179, 257–8
sexual abuse 160–1, 249
sexual domination 138, 141–2, 144–5
sexual harassment 138–9, 178–80
sexual objectification, of women 140
sexual violence, towards women 121, 123, 134, 138–42
sexual wellbeing 125–6
shame 43, 46, 58, 113, 118–19
Sharapova, Maria 122
shell shock 113
Showalter, Elaine 96, 104, 110, 113
Siddiqui, Hannana 140
Siedhoff, Matthew 227, 236–8, 249
Sims, J. Marion 298–9
Singh, Rama 61
Sjögren's syndrome 238, 265, 288–9
slavery 139, 298–9
sleep disturbance 69
Smith-Rosenberg, Carroll 98
social taboos *see* taboos
Society for Women's Health Research 295
Solnit, Rebecca 120–1
Sontag, Susan 198
sperm 50, 52, 65, 154
spontaneous desire 133
Srivastava, Ranjana 180, 182
Stamp, Nikki 7, 199–200
Steege, John 227, 236–8, 249
sterilisation 300–1

Stone, Louise 179–80
stoning, of women 137
suicide 178, 180, 182, 184, 261
Summers, Anne 141
surgeons 184
surgical menopause 65
Sydenham, Thomas 89–91
symptoms, dismissal of *see* medical
profession
systemic lupus erythematosus 285–7

taboos 10–12, 16, 21, 29–30, 42–3, 45–7,
104, 118, 127–8
Tait, Rachael 161, 174
'talking cure' 110–11
tampons 35–6, 43–4, 46
Tan, Caroline 179
Tarzian, Anita 233, 252
temporomandibular joint disorders
9–10, 225, 238–9, 270, *270*, 283
tension-type headache 10, 239, *270*,
278–9
testosterone 65, 70–1, 253–4
thyroid diseases 289–91
thyroiditis 285
transgender people 139, 253
Tyler Smith, W. 97

United Kingdom 43–4, 64, 73, 75, 140
United States 9–10, 44–6, 101–2, 139,
224, 257–8
Unwell (McRae) 80–1, 138, 300
urethra 35
Ussher, Jane 57–8, 71, 77, 113–14, 124,
140, 159–60
uterus 6, 12, 53, 86–9, 192, 243

vagina *22*, 28–31
vaginal dryness 69–70
vaginal mesh implants 154–7
vesicovaginal fistula 298–9
vestibulum 32, *33*, 35–6
victim blaming 159–60, 162, 198
Villarosa, Linda 257–8
Vincent, Katy 247, 250, 254, 314
Viner, Katharine 4
violence *see* family violence; sexual
violence, towards women
virginity 39–41
viscero-visceral hyperalgesia 244

vulva *22*, 29, 31–4, *33*
vulvodynia 9–10, 238–9, 245, 270, *270*,
273–4

Waller-Bridge, Phoebe 121
Watkins, Linda 229, 314
weight gain 68–9, 71
Weinhouse, Beth 297
wellness industry 320–1
Wenger, Nanette 14, 261
whales 76
Wier, Johannes 89
Williams, Naomi 206–11, 260
Williams, Serena 81–2, 122
Williams, Venus 122, 265
Willis, Thomas 89–91
Wilson, Robert 60, 71–3
witches 88–9
Wolf, Alli Sebastian 38
the womb *see* uterus
women
disadvantaged women 206–12
disparities in treatment of 15–17, 44,
176–7, 233–4, 252, 294–5
experiments on 298–302
as healers 99
historic duty of wives 140–1
ignorance about the body 11–12,
19–21, 28–9, 36, 118, 143
lack of knowledge of biology of 14,
177, 292–8, *293*
pelvic examinations without consent
301–2
prevalence of chronic pain 224–35
stereotypes of 12, 16, 50, 56, 176, 234,
252
unpaid labour of 44
at work 151
see also African-American women;
Indigenous women
Women's Health Institute (US) 72–3,
75, 310
women's health procedures 185–96
Wong, Kristina 121–2

Young, Kate 13, 45, 118, 153, 157,
167–8, 175, 177–8, 191, 195–7, 201,
292, 294–5, 301, 314, 320–1

Zucker, Irving 297